5/19

SPEECH AND
BRAIN-MECHANISMS

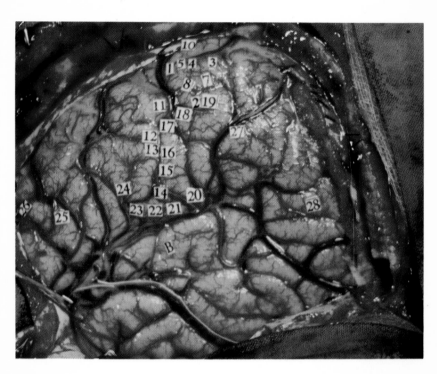

CASE C. H. Color photograph of the left hemisphere as exposed at operation. Application of electrode at points 26, 27 and 28 produced aphasic interference with speech. See page 111 for case description and Figure VII-5 for labelled drawing of brain.

SPEECH AND
BRAIN-MECHANISMS

BY WILDER PENFIELD AND
LAMAR ROBERTS

PRINCETON, NEW JERSEY
PRINCETON UNIVERSITY PRESS
1959

DR. WILDER PENFIELD has been Director of the
Montreal Neurological Institute since its found-
ing in 1934, and is Chairman of the Department
of Neurology and Neurosurgery of McGill University. He holds the Order of Merit from the
British Crown, and honorary degrees from 17
universities, including the two at which he was
once an undergraduate: Princeton and Oxford.

Among the learned societies of which he is a
fellow or member are the National Academy of
Sciences of the U.S. and of the U.S.S.R., the
Royal Society of London, the Académie Nationale
de Médecine, France, and the American Philosophical Society.

He has previously published six books on various phases of neurology, neurosurgery, and neurophysiology, and is at present working on an historical novel that deals with Hippocrates.

DR. LAMAR ROBERTS is Chief of Neurosurgery
at the University of Florida Medical School. After
earning his doctorate in medicine at Duke University, he was awarded the M.Sc. and Ph.D. degrees at McGill University for his graduate
studies on speech defects and neurological localization.

✧

Printed in the United States of America by
Princeton University Press, Princeton, New Jersey

Dedicated to

Helen Penfield and Louise Roberts

PREFACE

THIS book is the outcome of ten years of carefully planned study of brain dominance, and of aphasia and other speech disturbances. It is a discussion of the cerebral mechanisms of speech, the learning of language and the teaching of language.

During the ten year period of this study, the rapid flow of patients through an active Neurological Institute has brought us much useful material. And during that time a new method, mapping the limits of the cortical speech areas by electrical interference, has been developed. The use of the method and the study of a long series of cases of cortical excision, carried out for the treatment of focal epilepsy, has placed in our hands a remarkable body of evidence.

Our initial aim was to present this evidence in monograph form, together with a review of the literature. This we have done.

Our further intention was to make as clear a statement as we could of the neurophysiology of language and to locate its mechanisms. We have made a beginning on this second task. But hypothetical reasoning must always wait on the tests of time. And if, in the end, our hypotheses are found wanting, they should serve nonetheless to guide other explorers who pass this way.

Psychologists may well find as much useful material in this monograph as the clinicians and the neurophysiologists for whom it was originally intended. The fundamentals of speech mechanisms discussed here should help speech therapists.

The parts of this material suitable to a general university audience were used in the Vanuxem Lectures at Princeton University in 1956. That presentation modified inevitably the treatment of the evidence. Consequently a final chapter entitled *The Learning of Languages* has been added that may interest educators and the teachers of modern languages.

We have divided the writing of the chapters between us, and our initials are placed after each chapter heading to indicate the separate authorships. A Case Index will be found at the back of the book, as well as a General Index. Italics are used in the text to indicate the items that are placed in the General Index.

The initials A.D., that appear after Index and Case Index, are those of Miss Anne Dawson, Executive Secretary of the Montreal Neurological Institute. Her help and initiative in organizing the original materials during the years of study and her wise criticism of the manuscript give her a reasonable claim to a share in authorship.

There are many of our associates to whom we owe the deepest gratitude for the contributions they have made: Dr. Preston Robb, neurologist; Dr. Brenda Milner, psychologist; Professor Herbert Jasper, neurophysiologist; Professor Joseph Klingler, neuroanatomist; Miss Eleanor Sweezey, artist; Mr. Charles Hodge, photographer; and Mrs. Marion Casselman, typist-secretary.

Montreal
April, 1958   W.P. and L.R.

VANUXEM LECTURERS
AT PRINCETON UNIVERSITY

1912. Vito Volterra
1913. Emile Boutroux
1913. Arthur Denis Godley
1913. Alois Riehl
1913. Arthur Shipley
1914. Sir Walter Raleigh
1915. Thomas Hunt Morgan
1916. Charles Richard Van Hise
1917. Paul Elmer More
1918. H. H. Goddard
1919. Maurice De Wulf
1920. Henry A. Cotton
1921. Chauncey B. Tinker
1922. Vernon Kellogg
1923. A. J. B. Wace
1924. Louis T. More
1925. J. Franklin Jameson
1926. Henry Fairfield Osborn
1927. J. J. R. MacLeod
1928. A. N. Whitehead
1929. Sir James C. Irvine
1930. Bliss Perry
1931. Edwin P. Hubble
1932. Theobald Smith
1933. Archibald Bowman
1934. Herbert S. Jennings
1934. Frank Jewett Mather, Jr.
1935. Percy W. Bridgman
1936. Heinrich Bruening
1937. David Riesman
1938. Thomas Mann
1938. Detlev W. Bronk
1939. Earnest A. Hooton
1939. Francis G. Benedict
1940. Everette Lee DeGolyer
1941. George W. Corner
1942. William M. Stanley
1944. Edward Warner
1945. James B. Conant
1945. W. Albert Noyes
1945. Lee A. DuBridge

1945. A. Baird Hastings
1945. Walter S. Hunter
1945. Arthur H. Compton
1946. Patrick M. S. Blackett
1946. Herbert M. Evans
1946. Griffith C. Evans
1946. George Gaylord Simpson
1946. Percival C. Keith
1946. Frederic Charles Bartlett
1947. J. Robert Oppenheimer
1947. George W. Beadle
1948. Otto Struve
1948. Karl von Frisch
1948. Robert Broom
1949. Walter Bartky
1949. Lloyd Morris
1949. Dylan Thomas
1950. Julian Huxley
1950. Sir Richard Winn Livingstone
1950. Hermann Weyl
1950. Thomas Seward Lovering
1951. H. Munro Fox
1951. John R. Dunning
1951. Karl S. Lashley
1951. Dylan Thomas
1951. William Carlos Williams
1951. J. Allen Westrup
1952. Wolfgang Köhler
1952. George Gamow
1952. John von Neumann
1952. John E. Burchard
1952. Ralph Ellison
1953. George Wald
1953. Ernest Nagel
1954. Linus C. Pauling
1955. Konrad Lorenz
1956. Wilder Penfield
1956. H. P. Robertson
1957. Arend Heyting
1958. Claude Shannon
1958. Harold C. Urey

The general conclusions embodied in this monograph were presented by Wilder Penfield in the Vanuxem Lectures at Princeton University in February, 1956.

PREAMBLE TO THE
VANUXEM LECTURES

"The true function of knowledge is to be the servant of wisdom." In accordance with these words of Harold Dodds, President of Princeton University, my task in these Vanuxem Lectures is to draw from physiological facts some meaning that will serve the purposes of wisdom.

I came here years ago, and into this very Hall to be admitted to Princeton as a freshman. How well I remember it! I sat in one of those seats where you are sitting now and watched, through the lofty leaded windows, the leaves of an elm tree trembling against the blue of the sky, moving with the wind that none could feel. Unsuspected currents of the intellect must move, I thought, through Princeton. And I dreamed of the years to come.

How strange for me to stand here now, an old boy returning from his travels, returning home to tell a tale of how he listened to the humming of the mind's machinery, and where words come from.

W.P.

CONTENTS

CONTENTS

CONTENTS

SPEECH AND BRAIN-MECHANISMS

CHAPTER I

INTRODUCTION

W.P.

~~~~~~~~~~~~~~~~~~~~~~~~~~~~~~~~~~~~~~~

A. Prologue
B. Material
C. Brain activity—normal and epileptic
D. The messenger and the interpreter of
   consciousness
E. The brain and the mind

~~~~~~~~~~~~~~~~~~~~~~~~~~~~~~~~~~~~~~~

A. *Prologue*

THE general conclusions embodied in this monograph were presented in the 1956 Vanuxem Lectures. The audience at those lectures was drawn from the various departments of a great university. But most of the listeners had little familiarity with current work on the anatomy and physiology of the human brain. Consequently, the introduction was planned with this in mind. And now, since this book is designed for lay readers interested in speech mechanisms, as well as for the members of the medical profession, the same introduction will be used in this first chapter, with certain subtractions but without change in form.

The principal purpose of our study is to throw new light on the speech mechanisms of the brain—the mechanisms, for example, that enable me to speak to you and enable you to translate my words and understand my meaning. I select the words that are symbols of my thought. You, receiving these symbols, convert them into your own thought. But you hold short sequences of my words within the focus of your attention for a fleeting moment —long enough for conscious consideration—while you add your own interpretation. Then, letting that perception pass, you turn to the next sequence.

It is an astonishingly complex process that any speaker sets in motion. Consideration of it brings us, at once, face to face with the baffling problem of the nature of the *physical basis of the mind*. Without stopping for definition, let me say simply that I begin with what is called a thought. A succession of nerve impulses then flows out from my brain along the nerves in such a pattern that the appropriate muscles contract, while others relax, and I speak. An idea has found expression in electrical energy, movement, vibrations in the air. The boundary which separates philosophy from neurophysiology and physics has been crossed!

When that sound reaches your ear drums it is converted again into nerve impulses that are conducted along your auditory nerves and into your brain. This stream of nerve impulses results in a secondary mental proposition which resembles, but is far from being identical with, that of the speaker. It is a new perception. Again that strange *brain-mind frontier* has been crossed—crossed twice by each utterance!

Now, you may well wish to debate with me whether or not there is any boundary between nerve impulse and the mental state of a conscious person. And, furthermore, you might add that a neurophysiologist should confine his attention to neurone mechanisms, since he is only a physiologist after all. And yet in a discussion of speech he can hardly avoid consideration of this problem, and we shall return to it presently. Let me now get back on firmer ground where we can discuss the anatomy and physiology of the human brain briefly and simply.

B. *Material*

The material for these discussions is drawn from study of the patients in an active neurosurgical practice. During the past ten years my associate and co-author, Dr. Lamar Roberts, and I have been studying problems of speech and of brain dominance—a task to which I had turned somewhat earlier with the help of Dr. Preston Robb (1946).* Now Dr. Roberts has collected and reviewed all of the accumulated material.

Many patients came to us seeking a cure for *focal cerebral seizures* which had been caused by earlier injury, infection, or anoxia of the brain. The few who seemed suitable were selected for

---

* We owe much to our associates in the Montreal Neurological Institute. They have aided us in the organization of studies in clinical physiology. Particularly we thank Herbert Jasper, Professor of Experimental Neurology; Dr. Brenda Milner, clinical psychologist; and Mr. Robert Sparks, speech therapist. Most of all, we are indebted to the intelligent and forbearing patients who have helped us to understand many things in the operating room and out of it.

operation. The cases used in this sudy are chosen from that group.

Local anaesthesia was used during the operations (*osteoplastic craniotomy*). This does away with the pain of the procedure and yet leaves the brain normally active after a segment of the skull has been cut and temporarily turned back and the surface of the brain thus exposed. An operation is described in Chapter VII. Since the patients were talking and fully conscious during the procedures, it was possible to discover what parts of the cortex were devoted to the speech function.

We have reviewed 273 such operations upon the dominant hemisphere and an equal number on the opposite side for the purpose of this study, and Dr. Roberts has carried out a special series of speech examinations on seventy-two of the patients. The therapeutic purpose, in each case, was to remove areas of abnormal brain which were responsible for these attacks, without touching parts that were normal or too precious to be forfeited. Periodic *follow-up studies* show that such operations have stopped the attacks in about fifty per cent of the cases and made the attacks easier to control by medicine in others.

So much for clinical medicine. The problems of epilepsy and the anatomy and physiology of the human brain have been discussed elsewhere and our evidence summarized.* But it may serve a useful purpose to say a word here about activity in the normal brain and about the sudden abnormal activity that occurs from time to time in the brain of those who are subject to epileptic seizures.

C. *Brain activity—normal and epileptic*

The brain (Fig. III-1 on p. 40) is the convoluted organ which fills the great cavity of the skull. It is composed of *nerve cells* or *ganglion cells*, each provided with tail-like nerve fibers or expansions. Each living nerve cell is capable of developing energy that is propagated, as an electric current, along its own expansions. The expansions are insulated except at their endings. At the endings there are *synapses* across which enough energy can be communicated by a chemical process to the body of another nerve cell to fire off energy in it. Thus, further conduction of *electric potentials* passes through expansions of the second cell, and so by a

---

* Penfield and Rasmussen (1950); also Penfield and Jasper (1954).

succession of little activations a stream of impulses passes from one ganglion cell to another and another as determined, no doubt, by complicated facilitations and inhibitions.

It is said that there are ten billion nerve cells (ganglion cells) within the human brain, and each probably has some capacity of generating energy within itself. In addition to these there are even more neuroglial cells which seem to support and nourish and insulate the nerve cells and their branching fibers.

The business of the brain is carried out by the passage of nervous impulses from ganglion cell to ganglion cell in an orderly and controlled manner. The impulses pass quickly along the *insulated nerve fibers* like an electrical current, while passage across the synapses to successive nerve cells is accomplished by a somewhat slower chemical process. The cell bodies are collected together forming *gray matter,* and the nerve fibers which conduct the currents compose the *white matter.*

As long as the gray matter is normal, the energy of the nerve cells is employed only in the coordinated functional mechanisms of the brain. But if some area is injured by disease or pressure or lack of oxygen, the gray matter, although it may continue to function, may do so with abnormal additions of its own. There seems to be a defect in the regulating mechanisms which normally limit excessive discharge. Thus, sometimes months or years after injury, an abnormal area "ripens" slowly into a self-discharging electrochemical unit. This is called an *epileptogenic focus.*

In such an area or focus, excess electrical energy is formed and so, from time to time, unruly mass-discharges may be released. Such an explosive discharge produces an *epileptic fit.* The fit is large or small, depending upon the extent and intensity of discharge and the position of the gray matter involved. Consequently, the subject may suddenly make aimless movements over which he has no control, or he may have strange sensations or little dreams or memories. From one point of view these seizures are experiments carried out by disease upon the brain. As each attack unfolds, it may demonstrate to the watchful observer the position of the abnormality and also the functional uses of the area involved.

But (alas for the patient!) nature's experiment often turns into a grim tragedy. The attack, which begins as a small one, may spread to other areas and increase in severity until there is a maximum discharge. Then he has what people call an *epileptic fit*, a grand mal—falling unconscious with every muscle contracting, groaning, and perhaps frothing at the mouth. Thus, from earliest times epilepsy has been a curse to the epileptic. But when the discharge was small, nature's experiment has also been a teacher to observant physicians, and it still has much to teach us.

D. *The messenger and the interpreter of consciousness*

Hippocrates, the father of medicine, writing in the 5th century before Christ, made some thrilling observations on brain function. They are to be found in a medical lecture devoted to epilepsy. The affliction was then called the *sacred disease.**

Let Hippocrates' words set the stage for our discussion of the brain and the mind: "Some people say," he wrote, "that the heart is the organ with which we think, and that it feels pain and anxiety. But it is not so. . . . Men ought to know that from the brain and the brain alone, arise our pleasures, joys, laughter and jests, as well as our sorrows, pains, griefs and tears. Through it, in particular, we think, see, hear, and distinguish the ugly from the beautiful, the bad from the good, the pleasant from the unpleasant. . . . To consciousness the brain is the messenger. For when a man draws breath into himself, the air first reaches the brain, and so is dispersed through the rest of the body, though it leaves in the brain its quintessence, and all that it has of intelligence and sense. . . . Wherefore I assert that the brain is the *interpreter of consciousness.*"

You may quarrel with his conception of the way in which the brain takes energy from the air, but his reference to the brain-mind relation is magnificent. "To consciousness the brain is the messenger." And again, "The brain is the interpreter of consciousness." So it is with speech. To the speaker the brain becomes "the messenger," and for the listener the brain serves as the "interpreter." The message is a sequence of words.

---

* The Sacred Disease from Vol. II of Hippocrates, Loeb Classical Library, translated by W. H. S. Jones, 1952, p. 127 *et seq.*

E. *The brain and the mind*

It was pointed out above that if there is a frontier between mind and brain, it is crossed twice by each utterance during a lecture. Something seems to pass from the speaker's mind to his brain and from the listener's brain to his mind. That is assuming, of course, that the listener listens, and there is no assumption in the whole field of education that is so frequently false as this assumption!

In any case, when the listener does perceive the meaning of what is said, the record is laid down in some sort of ganglionic pattern—not the speaker's proposition necessarily, but the listener's perception of it. For a short time the listener can still reactivate his perception voluntarily. When he does so the frontier is crossed again. After a period of time it is forgotten—lost perhaps to voluntary recall. But the record remains there permanently, nonetheless, ready to be used as a flash-back for the purpose of comparison and interpretation. The nature of this *record of consciousness* and the mechanism of its re-employment will be discussed in Chapter III.

Let us consider the *brain-mind relationship* briefly. This is a problem to which a psychologist must turn his attention if he is concerned with psychology. It is a frontier toward which the religious thinker has made many an expedition, carrying with him a beloved guide-book. It is a boundary which, as some philosophers explain it, does not exist at all. But for the neurophysiologist there is a working boundary that does exist. Physiological methods bring him nearer and nearer to it. But he comes to an impasse, and beyond that impasse no present-day method can take him. If he should state that nerve impulses moving in certain patterns are one and the same thing as mind, he accomplishes little for his future work except to deprive himself of a useful working terminology.

Any man who adopts the dualistic terminology speaks of two elements in a living conscious human being: a body and a soul, a brain and a mind, electrical energy conducted through the *integrating pathways* of the cerebral hemispheres and *conscious thought*, a living machine and a spirit. However it is expressed, he must think either of a parallelism or a back and forth relationship.

The dualist believes that there is in each individual something additional to the body and its living energy. He may call it a conscious spirit which is the active accompaniment of brain activity and, thus, is present from birth to death except, perhaps, in states of deep sleep and coma. He may also believe that this spirit continues its existence after the death of the body, and that it is somehow one with God. By such belief, he extends the dualism of the individual to a dualism of the universe. The time has passed when the church need necessarily look upon intellectualism as hostile to faith.

These concepts of the spirit, and of God, are the things a scientist may believe. But it is what has been called an act of faith. He may organize his life and his work accordingly. But, whatever his inward belief may be, he must recognize that there are no methods in science by which he can test or verify these hypotheses, and that, therefore, his faith in such matters carries with it no greater stamp of authority than that of any other thinking person in any other walk of life.

The need, which many scientists feel, of working with the dual concepts of mind and body was expressed by the distinguished anatomist C. Judson Herrick (1955) as follows:

"The mind-body problem," he wrote, "will never be solved by ignoring the troublesome factors, either those of spirit or of matter. The enquiry cannot be limited to either the conscious or the unconscious factors, because what we are looking for is the relation between the two. . . . Traditional materialism (the 'crude' variety) and classical spiritualism (or, more reputably, 'idealism') both involve neglect of a vast wealth of human experience, including common sense and refined scientific knowledge. We cannot choose between materialism and spiritualism. We must have both."

But two other general hypotheses have been employed: First, there is the point of view, once so persuasively taught by Bishop Berkley, that matter does not exist except insofar as it is conceived in the mind of man or in the mind of God.

Secondly, there is the contrary point of view described as materialism. For those who adhere to this belief, there is no spirit, and the mind of man is to be explained completely by the mechanisms of the brain.

More recently there is a third approach to this matter—a

philosophical approach—which was expressed by Gilbert Ryle (1950) as follows: "The umbrella-titles of 'Mind' and 'Matter' obliterate the very differences that ought to interest us. Theorists should drop both these words. 'Mind' and 'Matter' are echoes from the hustings of philosophy, and prejudice the solutions of all problems posed in terms of them."

The pupils of Ivan Pavlov hope that the conditioned reflexes, which he showed to be so important in some of the learning processes of animals, may yet serve the purposes of a materialistic explanation of the mind. The conditioned reflex enables the animal to adjust to its environment, in part at least, and it is obvious that this would be consistent with the philosophy of Marx, so popular in the Soviet Union today. It is interesting that at present, a most important part of the research of physiologists in that country is devoted to conditioned reflexes. It is good work but the problem is not yet solved.

Perhaps, as Lord Adrian has pointed out, the difficulty will eventually be "solved by some enlargement of the boundaries of natural science" and the appearance of a new psychology.

We are trying to create that enlargement today, but we must not be too impatient in our desire to complete the quest. After all, it is the "revelation of the mystery which was kept secret since the world began"* that we are seeking.

Aristotle pointed out the inconsistency of psychologists in the 4th century B.C., saying, "They place the soul in the body and attach it to the body without trying in addition to determine the reason why, or the condition of the body under which such attachment is produced."†

Theorists, as Ryle proposes, may be able to give up a dualistic terminology. But biologists are not theorists. And there is no place in scientific medicine for the unprovable hypothesis. We must be content to study man and animal by the scientific method, using the language of "busy common sense." This is the language of dualism.

We have at present no basis for a scientific explanation of the *brain-mind relationship*. We can only continue to study the brain without philosophical prejudice. And if the day should ever dawn

* Romans 16:25.
† *De Anima I* 3, 22-23 (Wallace translation).

when scientific analysis of body and brain solves the "mystery," all men who have sought the truth in all sincerity will rejoice alike: the professing materialist and the dualist, the scientist and the philosopher, the agnostic and the convinced worshipper. Surely none need fear the truth.

CHAPTER II

FUNCTIONAL ORGANIZATION OF THE HUMAN BRAIN, DISCRIMINATIVE SENSATION, VOLUNTARY MOVEMENT

W.P.

~~~~~~

A. The organ of the mind
B. Parts of the central nervous system
C. The cerebrum
D. Centrencephalic integration
E. Some functional subdivisions of the cortex
   1. Primary motor and sensory transmitting areas
   2. Secondary and supplementary areas
   3. Subdivision of cerebral cortex by means of stimulation

~~~~~~

THE Sumerians and the Babylonians looked upon the liver as the seat of the intellect, while Hebrews from Genesis to the Acts of the Apostles referred to the heart as the dwelling place of mind and spirit. Thus, when an Arab today refers to a friend as the joy of his liver, there is good historical background for the expression. Men in other lands, using many different tongues, still speak of the heart's desire, and they take to heart life's most profound lessons to ponder them there.

It was pointed out in the Introduction that even four hundred years before Christ, Hippocrates knew that the brain was the organ with which men thought. He was aware of the fact that injury to one hemisphere of the brain might produce paralysis of the arm and leg on the other side. This indicated some degree of localization of function. But his opinions found little acceptance and they were subsequently ignored. There seems to have been no serious consideration of subdivisions of functional areas within the brain until 1861, when Paul Broca pointed out that there was an area in the brain specially devoted to speech.

12

A. *The organ of the mind*

At the beginning of the 19th century the accepted teaching was simply that the brain was the organ of the mind. But it operated, as a whole, like other organs—the liver, for example, and the heart. Men spoke of the brain as children speak of a clock, saying, "It tells the time"—children who have not yet looked into the works.

At the beginning of the century phrenologists, led by Gall and Spurzheim in Vienna, were placing their hands upon men's skulls and drawing fantastic conclusions. They subdivided the great organ inside the head into little organs. In the little organs there were, they said, representations of different feelings and intellectual faculties such as love of children, sexual passion, acquisitiveness, benevolence, wit, language.

The more orthodox teachers in the Universities ridiculed this first effort by medical "quacks" to introduce a conception of functional localization. But academicians and phrenologists alike were making the mistake that still haunts our thinking on this subject. The former said function dwells in the brain as a whole. The latter said separate functions dwelt in separate compartments, operating as autonomous units.

This misconception lingers on in the minds of modern neurophysiologists and clinicians. It is so easy to say that the "representation" of movement is here and sensation is there in the cerebral cortex, as though such things could have independent dwelling places.

At about the same time that Gall and Spurzheim were publishing their treatise on phrenology (they gave it the presumptuous title of "The Anatomy and Physiology of the Nervous System"!), the first steps toward an explanation of the working of the brain were being made in Italy. It was then that Galvani and Volta were initiating the study of electricity and the conduction of electrical currents along nerves.

The illuminating discovery by the French surgeon, Paul Broca, was that a patient had lost the power of speech without other serious defect. He showed the cause at autopsy: a restricted lesion in the left hemisphere of the brain. It was located in the general region of the third frontal convolution. That clinical observation in 1861 was of great importance in the history of neurology.

The next momentous event came when Fritsch and Hitzig (1870) applied an electric current to the cerebral cortex of a lightly anaesthetized dog. The limbs on the opposite side of the body moved. Here, under the experimenter's electrode, was the place of movement control—a place, they thought, where mind might enter body.

Let us consider the clock again. It is not enough to recognize that the second hand, the hour hand, and the chimes all have partially separable mechanisms of their own, and that the chimes, for example, may be paralyzed without stopping the hands. He who would understand the clock-works must analyze the interrelationship of its mechanisms and the transmission of forces that makes the clock tell time.

Today we are beginning to see into the works within the head. We perceive that the secret of functional activity in the living brain is the movement within it of "transient electrical potentials, travelling the fibers of the nervous system" (Sherrington's phrase). We surmise that it is the changing pattern of these travelling potentials, as they flash into this or that portion of the total mechanism, that makes possible the ever-changing content of the mind.

It is now almost a century since Broca showed that speech had some degree of neuronal localization in the brain. He demonstrated that what he called *aphemia,* and what we now call *aphasia,* was produced by a relatively small destruction of a certain area of cortex in the dominant hemisphere of a man. This meant, of course, not that speech was located there in the sense of a phrenologist's localization, but that the area in question was used as an essential part of a functional mechanism employed while the individual spoke, wrote, read, or listened to others who spoke. It showed further that a man could still think and carry out other forms of voluntary activity while the speech mechanism was paralyzed. The clock still ran, although the chimes had been silenced.

B. *Parts of the central nervous system*

In recent decades, the action of the brain has been analyzed with great industry, and parts of its many integral functions have been mapped out. For those who are unfamiliar with this field, a preliminary discussion of some present concepts of the physiology of the central nervous system of man may serve the purposes of orientation. Chapters II and III will be devoted to this purpose, and in Chapter X we will reconsider our observations on speech mechanisms against this background.

Some portions of the human central nervous system are outlined in Figure II-1. The spinal cord contains primitive reflex arcs

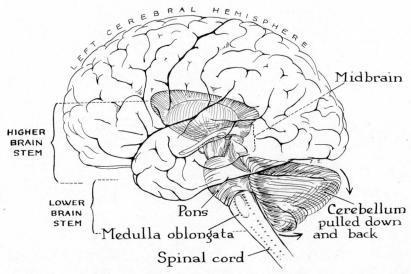

FIG. II-1. The central nervous system of man. The higher brain stem, including thalamus, midbrain, and part of pons are shown within the brain. The lower brain stem composed of pons and medulla emerges below with the cerebellum.

related to muscle movement and tone. The medulla oblongata, at the upper end of the cord, contains the primary reflex mechanisms of respiration as well as cardiovascular and gastro-intestinal reflexes. The cerebellum is the head ganglion of the proprioceptive system. It receives information from the vestibular labyrinths regarding body position and movement, and from the muscles as to their position and movement. It influences muscle tone and coordinates the movements which may be initiated elsewhere in the central nervous system.

The cerebral hemispheres, taken together with the higher brain stem that unites them, are related to these activities and also to acquired reactions, voluntary activities, and states of consciousness. The midbrain is well named since it plays an intermediary role. Together with the adjacent brain stem below, it contains centers for reflex regulation of muscle tone and body posture and movement. Thus it has a close functional relationship to the cerebellum and pons, medulla, and cord below it. But it is also oriented in the other direction. It includes an important part of the brain stem reticular system, and it provides neuronal mechanisms which seem to be essential to consciousness and the integration of function in the cerebral hemispheres.

It is not possible to point to any sharp functional frontier. There are no sharp functional levels between the higher brain stem, which includes the thalamus, and the lower brain stem which is primarily involved in the coordination of more primitive activities. Nevertheless, it is of interest to consider the result of transection through the midbrain. When an anaesthetic is given to a cat, for example, the cerebrum seems to be "put to sleep," and so the animal is unconscious. If, then, a transection is made at the upper level of the midbrain and the cerebrum is thus removed, the animal does not wake up when the anaesthetic is withdrawn. It has become a decerebrate animal—an automatic motor mechanism. Sherrington showed that the decerebrate "preparation" could be "touched" into action in certain ways. It pulled its limb away from the thorn that pricked it. Milk in the mouth was swallowed; acid was rejected. It might stand and even walk a little, might vocalize and even purr.

But the decerebrate animal has no "thoughts, feelings, memory, percepts, conations." It moves and adjusts to an immediate environment. "The mindless body reacts with the fatality of a multiple penny-in-the-slot machine to certain stimuli."* It is an *automaton* that seems to satisfy the conception of the most exacting materialist.

* The quotations are from Sir Charles Sherrington. Bazett and Penfield (1922) showed that the "chronic decerebrate preparation," kept alive for weeks, maintained the general characteristics described by Sherrington in the decerebrate animal during the shorter experiments that he carried out.

C. *The cerebrum*

"It is then around the cerebrum, its physiological and psychological attributes, that the main interest of biology must ultimately turn."* The mammal's brain, in contradistinction to its lower brain stem, cerebellum, and spinal cord, has evolved with the distance receptors: the organs of smell, vision, and hearing. To some extent, the hemispheres are built upon the distance receptors. But in the case of man, as contrasted with other animals, vast new additional areas of cerebral cortex have made their appearance, crowding the sensory and the motor areas of the cortex down into the deep fissures. His olfactory areas, which bulk so large in the brain of lower animals, have shrunk to a position of negligible importance in olfactory bulb and temporal lobe.

There remain three important sensory areas in the human cortex (Fig. II-2 and Fig. II-5), which receive projected streams of nerve impulses as follows: 1) from the eyes, through lateral geniculate nuclei, to the primary visual sensory areas about each calcarine fissure on the mesial surfaces of each occipital lobe (see also Fig. II-9); 2) from the ears to the buried transverse gyri of Heschl, which form part of the first temporal convolution on each side and run deep into the lateral fissure of Sylvius; 3) from face, arm, leg, and body to the somatic sensory areas in the postcentral gyrus of each side.

There are also the primary somatic motor areas (Fig. II-2 and Fig. II-5), one in each hemisphere, which pass on the streams of nerve impulses that are projected downward through the ganglionic junctions in medulla and spinal cord to the muscles of face, limbs, and body. These outflowing impulses, thus, produce the action we call voluntary.

These are the four major areas of cortex that have what may be called trunk lines of communications through to the outside world (Cobb, 1944). Three bring in information; one sends out the stream of impulses that determines voluntary action, an important part of which is talking and writing.

Removal of the calcarine area of one occipital lobe produces

* This was the final sentence written by Sherrington in his Silliman Lectures, delivered at Yale University in 1904, and published as "The Integrative Action of the Nervous System." Scribners, New York, 1906.

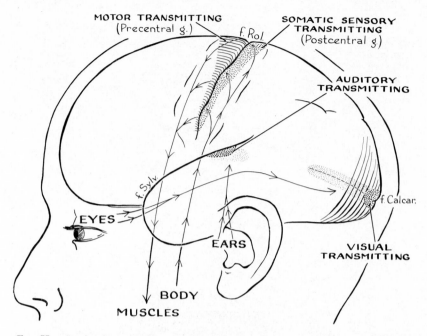

Fig. II-2. Projection areas of cortex. *Transmitting areas* on the lines of communication with environment. Three important sensory transmitting areas (stippled) pass afferent informative streams of impulses through the cerebral cortex to brain stem. The voluntary motor system carries impulses in a planned pattern through the motor transmitting area (lined) on the precentral gyrus, out to the muscles that control voluntary movement. The functional contribution of the cortex to the sensory and motor streams that pass through it is not clear.

blindness in the opposite field of vision. Removal of one postcentral gyrus results in loss of discriminatory sensation from the opposite side of the body. Removal of one transverse gyrus of Heschl, on the other hand, affects hearing little, if at all, perhaps because the incoming auditory impulses pass from each ear to both auditory areas. Removal of the precentral gyrus results in permanent paralysis of skilled or delicate movements in the opposite hand and the foot. But voluntary movement of the proximal joints of arm and leg are not lost, and there is no more than a minor interference with movement of face and mouth after cortical removal of face area.

It must be added that there are additional motor and sensory areas (see Fig. II-10). The supplementary motor area projects its impulses, outside the brain, down the spinal cord also (Bertrand, 1956). There is also a second somatic sensory area which receives impulses directly from the periphery. There are also secondary visual areas which surround the primary calcarine fissure. These secondary and supplementary areas can be removed, at least on one side, with little or no resultant deficit. There is also a probable secondary auditory area adjacent to the primary auditory area. The vestibular areas may well be nearby.

The other vast areas of the human cortex, such as those in the temporal, the anterior frontal, and the posterior parietal lobes, have connections within the brain itself which enable them to carry out functions that may be described as psychical rather than sensory or motor. But all areas of cortex are united with sub-cortical gray matter by means of two-way specific or non specific nerve fiber projection systems* (see Fig. II-3).

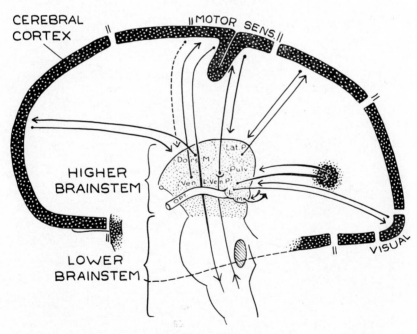

Fig. II-3. Diagram of connections between brain stem and cerebral cortex corresponding with Fig. II-4. This illustrates the hypothesis that each functional area of cortex forms a unit with some portion of the diencephalon of which it is the developmental projection. After Penfield and Jasper, 1954.

* Jasper: Subcortical Interrelationships, Chapter IV of Penfield and Jasper, 1954.

D. *Centrencephalic integration*

It has long been assumed that the cerebral cortex was the summit, functionally speaking, and that the business of the mind was somehow transacted there. The transactions were somehow to be carried out there by means of "association" areas of cortex and the transcortical fiber systems. According to this conception, the visual information that came from the right half of the visual field to the left hemisphere would have to be made available across the hemisphere to the precentral gyrus, so that appropriately patterned impulses could be sent out to the right hand. But what about the other hand, and the other field of vision, and what about the plan of action?

It is obvious that the brain must have a central coordinating and integrating mechanism. If this "machine" is at all like other machines, there must be a place toward which streams of sensory impulses converge. There must be a place from which streams of motor impulses emerge to move the two hands in simultaneous, planned action. There must be neuronal circuits in which activity of both hemispheres is somehow summarized and fused—circuits the activation of which makes conscious planning possible.

From certain philosophical points of view the foregoing assumption might be denied at once. Since no one knows the nature of mental activity, it is as easy to conceive of it in relation to the surface of the two hemispheres in simultaneous neuronal action (and even in the peripheral nerves too) as it is to believe that it depends on a centrally placed zone of neurone circuits where neuronal activity is summarized and finally integrated.

But a neurophysiologist may not listen to such objections, especially when the evidence before him seems to indicate that such central integration is actually taking place. And a clinician, who is forced to take action in order to deal with patients, must construct a working hypothesis.

In 1936, in a paper entitled "The cerebral cortex and consciousness,"* the clinical evidence was examined with the following conclusion:

There is "evidence of a level of integration within the central nervous system that is higher than that to be found in the cerebral

* The Harvey Lecture, New York Academy of Medicine, Penfield, 1938.

cortex." There is a "regional localization of the neuronal mechanism involved in this integration" which is "most intimately associated with the initiation of voluntary activity and with the sensory summation prerequisite to it. . . . All regions of the brain may well be involved in normal conscious processes, but the indispensable substratum of consciousness lies outside the cerebral cortex, . . . not in the new brain but in the old . . . probably in the diencephalon."

In 1946 it was pointed out* in a paper on "Highest Level Seizures" that Hughlings Jackson's "highest level" of integration was located not in the frontal lobes, as he had suggested, but "in the diencephalon and mesencephalon."

In 1950, in a report on "Epileptic automatism and centrencephalic integrating system" (Penfield, 1952), it was proposed that, because of criticism of the term "highest level" as suggesting separation of one level from another, the word "centrencephalic" might be used to identify that system within diencephalon, mesencephalon, and probably rhombencephalon, which has bilateral functional connections with cerebral hemispheres. "The *centrencephalic system*" was then defined as "that central system within the brain stem which has been, or may be in the future, demonstrated as responsible for integration of the function of the hemispheres."†

It has been suggested by our associate, Professor Herbert Jasper, that the definition should be enlarged to include "integration of varied specific functions from different parts of one hemisphere." We are forced to agree with him. The subcortical coordinating centers which will be described for speech in this monograph are integrating areas within one hemisphere. Thus, although the centrencephalic system would not include the cranial nerve nuclei of the brain stem, it would include all those areas of subcortical gray matter (together with their connecting tracts) which serve the purposes of inter-hemispheral integration and intra-hemispheral integration.‡

* Penfield and Jasper, 1947. Hughlings Jackson (1890) described "highest level fits" in his Lumelian Lectures.

† The brain stem, as defined by Herrick, includes the thalamus on either side but not the cerebellum nor the cerebral cortex and their dependencies.

‡ It would seem that the corpus striatum, or basal mass of gray and white matter in each hemisphere, forms an extra-pyramidal motor mechanism and is probably not to be considered a part of the higher centrencephalic integrating system.

For the past twenty years this hypothesis has been tested by practical application in the problems of patients crowding through the Montreal Neurological Institute—men and women, conscious and unconscious, with lesions and local epileptic discharges in many different areas, patients seen in the consulting room, in the operating room, and also, alas, in the autopsy room. This experience taken with evidence from many other sources* seems to leave no other hypothesis tenable and establishes it as a working theory. The brilliant work of Morison, Magoun, Jasper, and many others on the reticular system with its "non specific" connections is a most important beginning of anatomical confirmation.

We will continue to assume, therefore, that there is a central integrating system situated within the higher brain stem. Integration reaches the highest level there, in the sense of Jacksonian philosophy, but it is presumably never divorced from the activity of some areas of the cortex and especially certain areas of the temporal lobes and the anterior portions of the frontal cortex.

Under normal circumstances, consciousness accompanies this combined activity. Consciousness disappears with interruption of function in the centrencephalic system.

Bits of evidence which support this thesis are many. Any area of cortex may be removed on either side without loss of consciousness. All areas except those devoted to speech have been removed in our clinic at one time or another during the treatment of focal cortical epilepsy or for the control of involuntary movements. Whether or not the centrencephalic system could function at all, if all areas of cortex could be removed at once in a single individual, is a question which cannot be answered. It must remain a matter of speculation as to the way in which the subject would still be considered "conscious." On the other hand, any lesion, such as a tumor exerting pressure or some agent that interferes with the circulation in the higher brain stem, is accompanied by unconsciousness.

* Our very great indebtedness to other writers and associates is acknowledged in other publications, e.g. Penfield and Rasmussen, 1950; Penfield and Jasper, 1954; etc. The attempt in this monograph to present neurophysiological concepts to those who have little experience in the field might well be defeated if it bristled with such references.

E. *Some functional subdivisions of the cortex*

Each functional subdivision of the cerebral cortex of man may be looked upon as an outgrowth or projection outward of some area of gray matter in the older brain stem (Fig. II-4). Thus, the projected area in the newly formed cortex presumably serves to amplify and enlarge a function already being served in some sort of rudimentary manner by the old brain of more elementary animals.

For example, the anterior frontal cortex might be thought of as an elaboration from the dorso-medial nucleus of the thalamus, and much of the temporal cortex as an outward projection of the pulvinar and posterior part of the lateral nucleus of the thalamus (Fig. II-3). This is in many ways a surer guide by which to predict functional subdivision than the cyto-architectonic parcellation of cortex (e.g. Brodmann's areas, Fig. II-5).

As a preliminary to our discussion of speech it may serve a useful purpose to describe in general outline some of the functional areas of the cerebral cortex of man. These areas have been determined largely by electrical stimulation and by operative excision. The areas thus determined are sensory or motor or psychical.

1. *Primary motor and sensory transmitting areas*

The primary *motor transmitting area* of the cerebral cortex is situated on the precentral gyrus largely within the central fissure of Rolando. Part of the cortico-spinal tracts take origin here. But the stream of neuronal impulses that produces voluntary activity does not originate in the cortex. It comes from a subcortical source (Penfield, 1954a). That this is so is supported by the fact that excision of the convolutions immediately in front of or behind the gyrus does not prevent a patient from controlling the contralateral hand and guiding it according to many sources of information (Fig. II-6). He can still direct the movement of this hand in accordance with visual information that enters the brain through the visual area in the occipital lobe of that side. Indeed, if the occipital lobe is amputated, he can still direct the hand, thanks to

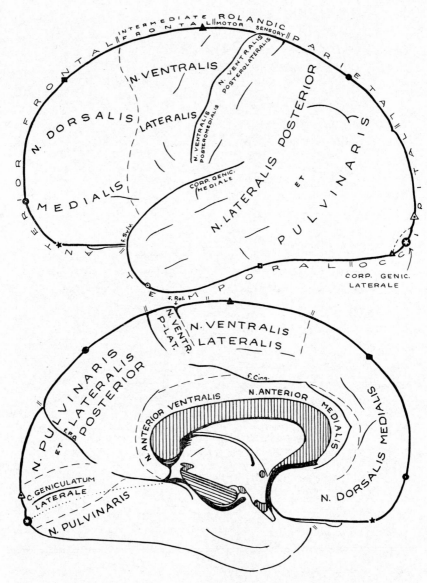

Fig. II-4. Projection of nuclear masses of the thalamus and geniculate bodies out to the cerebral cortex, as suggested by the thalamo-cortical connections. This is based on the work of Earl Walker (1938a, 1938b). Lateral surface above, mesial surface below. From Penfield and Jasper, 1954.

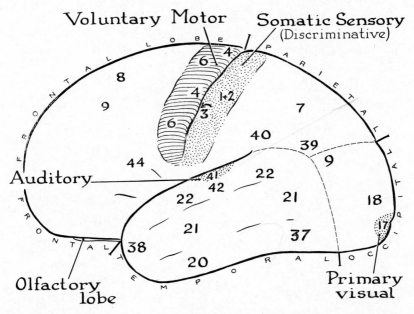

FIG. II-5. Left hemisphere with some of Brodmann's architectonic cortical subdivisions shown by numbers. The lobes are indicated as are some of the cortical transmitting stations for sensation and voluntary movement. Taste and visceral sensation, which have stations deep in the fissure of Sylvius and on the insula, are not indicated. Vestibular sensation, which probably has some cortical allotment near to the auditory area, is not shown. Most of the auditory area is buried in the fissure of Sylvius; most of the primary visual area, in the calcarine fissure; and the somatic area for discriminative sensation, within the central fissure of Rolando. The tracts which serve pain sensation are not shown; they end in the thalamus and make no essential detour to the cortex like those of the other forms of sensation.

the visual impulses that are entering the brain through the other occipital lobe.

Therefore, it seems reasonable to assume that the stream of impulses (broken line in Fig. II-7) which, by its pattern, determines how the hand is to move, must originate in a ganglionic area of the centrencephalic system. And since the hands are used so much together, it seems likely that the ganglionic area is intimately related to the source of the stream of impulses that is flowing in the other direction out to the motor area devoted to hand control in the other hemisphere.

The motor area of the cortex is therefore an arrival platform and a departure platform (Fig. II-7). Its function is to transmit

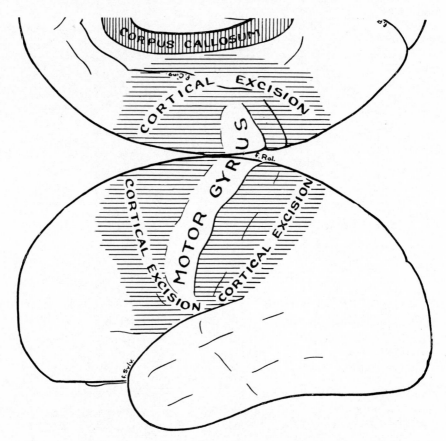

FIG. II-6. Diagram to show the areas (lined) adjacent to the precentral gyrus, in which surgical excision does not deprive a man of capacity for voluntary movement by making use of the various sources of sensory information entering the brain through both hemispheres.

and possibly to transmute, with the aid of secondary motor areas, the patterned stream of impulses which arises in the centrencephalic system and passes on out to the target in voluntary muscles. There is, therefore, a supra-cortical or pre-cortical portion of the voluntary motor pathway and an infra-cortical or post-cortical portion, with a motor-transmitting strip of cortex uniting them.

The somatic sensory area on the postcentral gyrus likewise is a transmitting strip. Excision of cortex posterior to it, or even of the precentral gyrus anterior to it, does not deprive the patient of the information which normally reaches this arrival platform. The

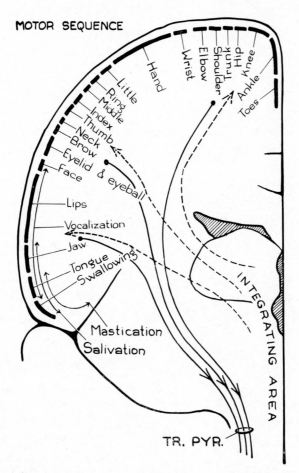

FIG. II-7. Voluntary motor tracts. Cross-section through right hemisphere along the plane of the precentral gyrus. The pathway of control of voluntary movement is suggested from gray matter, somewhere in the higher brain stem, by the broken lines to the motor transmitting strip of the precentral gyrus. From there it runs down the cortico-spinal tract, as shown by the unbroken lines toward the muscles. The sequence of responses to electrical stimulation on the surface of the cortex (from above down, along the motor strip from toes through arm and face to swallowing) is unvaried from one individual to another. From Penfield and Jasper, 1954.

somatic sensory stream which comes in from the skin, muscles, and joints of the body goes to the postcentral gyrus (Fig. II-8), after ganglionic interruption in the lateral nucleus of the thalamus. But it must, therefore, return inward to join the centrencephalic system along a post-cortical limb (broken line in Fig. II-8).

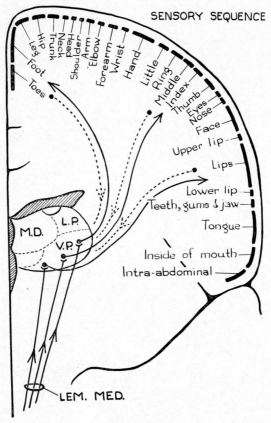

Fig. II-8. Somatic sensation. Cross-section of the left hemisphere along the plane of the postcentral gyrus. The afferent pathway for discriminative somatic sensation is indicated by the unbroken lines coming up, through the medial lemniscus, to the transmitting strip on the postcentral gyrus, and from there on by the broken lines into the centrencephalic circuits of integration. There is, no doubt, close inter-relationship between sensory and motor activity of the units shown in this Figure and the preceding one, across the central fissure. From Penfield and Jasper, 1954.

Something similar may be said of the primary *visual area* of the cortex. It is located on the banks of the calcarine fissure situated in the mesial surface of the occipital lobe (Fig. II-9). Removal of the area produces complete blindness in the opposite visual field (homonymous hemianopsia) except perhaps for the small half disc of central vision. This disc at the center of the field of vision sends its afferent stream (it is claimed by some investigators) through the visual area of the ipsilateral cortex as well as the contralateral.

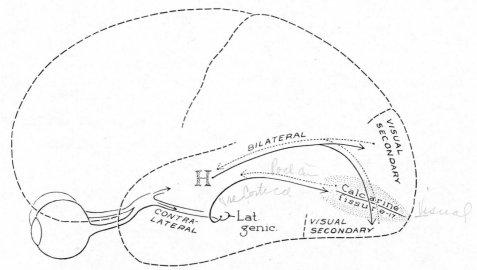

Fig. II-9. Diagram of pathway of visual sensory afferent impulses from the left side of the retina of each eye to the transmitting cortex of the calcarine fissure of the left hemisphere, and then onward as suggested by the broken line into the circuits of integration. The left calcarine transmitting cortex receives information only from the right homonymous field, except perhaps in the small zone about the point of central visual fixation where, some say, both fields find representation. The secondary visual area has a relation to both visual fields. The stippled letter H indicates subcortical areas of intercommunication and integration.

Removal of adjacent occipital cortex, if the primary calcarine area is spared, does not produce blindness in the contralateral field and does not make it difficult for the patient to guide his hands or feet in accordance with what he sees in that field.

Consequently, it is evident that the primary visual sensory area of each hemisphere is a visual transmitting area. The visual pathway, from eye to centrencephalic system, may also be divided into a pre-cortical and a post-cortical portion. In Figure II-9 the pre-cortical limb is a black line and the post-cortical limb, a broken line.

The rest of the cortex that makes up each occipital lobe may be called a secondary visual area. Its removal does not produce hemianopsia but electrical stimulation there, just as in the primary area, causes a conscious patient to see colors, lights, stars, shadows. All of the secondary sensory areas seem to be relatively dispensable. They will be discussed in a subsequent section.

By analogy, the auditory cortex on Heschl's transverse gyri of each hemisphere is likewise a transmitting area—a way station in the stream of auditory impulses.

If these three important sensory areas (for somatic, visual, and auditory information) are used for nothing more than transmission, then the question follows: Why do these streams of sensory impulses make such a detour to the cortex after their synaptic interruption in the lateral nucleus of the thalamus? Furthermore, why should the voluntary motor pathway make a cortical detour?

These questions are clearly unscientific, since they are based on teleological thinking, on the assumption that all such arrangements have their purpose. Nevertheless, the questions deserve consideration, especially since no final answer can be given at the present!

First of all it must be stated clearly that, although the sensory and motor currents flow through the corresponding areas of cortex to more distant goals, it is quite possible that highly important transmutations in those currents are brought about in the cortex, and that the transcortical relationships, which the primary areas maintain with secondary sensory and motor areas and other more distant areas, may be of great importance. The same may be said of the inter-hemispheral commissures such as the corpus callosum.

The surface area of each primary sensory area in the cortex is relatively great, as compared with the ganglionic area allotted to it in the higher brain stem. For example, in the case of vision, the calcarine cortex is considerably more extensive than the lateral geniculate ganglion. It is quite possible that each transmitting platform is used to sort out the elements in the stream of arriving impulses and so sends on a reorganized stream of impulses.

Perhaps the voluminous secondary sensory cortex which borders each of the primary areas contributes to this task. Perhaps, also, the fact that the interpretive cortex and speech cortex, which we shall describe shortly, lie as they do between the secondary visual and secondary auditory cortex, makes possible other types of *transcortical functional communications*.

The same answer might be given to the question regarding the motor transmitting area (Brodmann's area 4) on the precentral gyrus. Perhaps the cortex of this gyrus somehow reorganizes the stream in its passage onward to bulb and spinal cord. And the supplementary motor area may well add something, and also the closely connected somatic sensory areas of the postcentral gyrus. But all such discussions of transcortical functional activity are, at present, no more than surmise.

2. Secondary and supplementary areas*

The secondary and supplementary areas are shown in part in Figure II-10. The whole of the precentral gyrus (Brodmann's area 6 as well as 4) is called primary for the purpose of this discussion; and the whole of the postcentral gyrus likewise, although subdivisions of each gyrus into primary and secondary might be attempted. The calcarine cortex is considered primary. In man we have no evidence, as yet, that would differentiate primary from secondary in the auditory cortex, although this has been done suggestively for the laboratory mammals.

As an example of the distinction between primary and secondary, let us take the occipital lobe: Stimulation of Brodmann's area 17 (Fig. II-5), which forms the banks of the calcarine fissure, causes the patient to see lights, shadows, colors, usually moving or twinkling in the opposite visual field. The rest of the occipital lobe is made up of Brodmann's area 18 and 19, and stimulation there produces the same types of visual phenomena, but the lights and colors may appear to the patient to be in either visual field. Excisions restricted to the secondary visual cortex do not produce homonymous hemianopsia.

Furthermore, stimulation of the second somatic sensory area (Fig. II-10) causes the patient to feel sensations usually, though not always, similar to those produced in the postcentral gyrus. Thus he feels a tingling, numbness, sense of movement, desire to move. But, whereas application of the electrode to the postcentral gyrus in arm or leg areas produces contralateral sensation only, application to the *second sensory area* within the fissure of Sylvius occasionally produces ipsilateral and bilateral instead of contralateral sensation. Removal of second sensory areas of cortex produces no obvious sensory or motor defect.

---

* The terms secondary and supplementary are used here to designate areas of cortex which give rise to sensation or movement on stimulation but which on removal do not abolish capacity to see or feel or move.

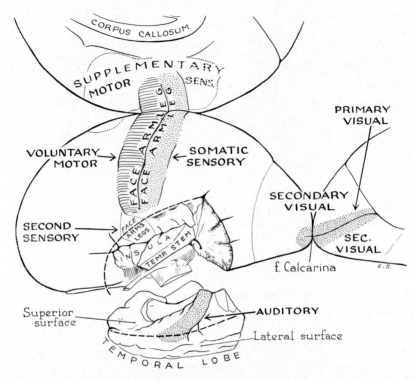

FIG. II-10. Primary transmitting areas (sensory: dotted, and motor: lined) and some secondary sensory and motor areas in the cortex of the left hemisphere. Parts of the mesial surfaces are shown. The temporal lobe is cut and turned down to expose its superior surface (which is ordinarily hidden in the fissure of Sylvius) and the primary auditory area on the transverse gyrus of Heschl. No secondary auditory area is figured, since our stimulation evidence is not sufficient to establish its limits in man. The extent of second sensory (somatic) area is probably greater than that shown on the upper Sylvian bank. The sensory responses in the posterior portion of the supplementary somatic areas have, as yet, been few in number, but the motor responses have been numerous and easily elicited.

And finally, excision of one *supplementary motor area* seems to produce no more functional defect than a decrease in capacity for speed of rapidly alternating movement of hand and foot. Stimulation of the supplementary area causes the patient to make turning and postural movements that employ both sides of the body—movements which the conscious patient is quite helpless to resist.

The relationship between the primary areas of transmitting

cortex and the secondary areas might be illustrated by a consideration of the organization of vision shown in the hypothetical drawing of Figure II-9. Here, it is suggested that the secondary areas
receive impulses from both fields of vision. Thus the secondary
area would be receiving an almost instantaneous echo of the information that has entered the brain through the transmitting
apparatus of both sides.

Whatever the true function of the secondary and supplementary
sensory and motor areas of the cortex may be, it is obvious that
there would be no room for these large areas of gray matter in the
older brain stem. Increased allotment of space came to each of
these functional systems because of the cortical detours. This
applies to mammals in general and especially to man.

3. Subdivision of the cerebral cortex
by means of stimulation

It was in 1870 that an electrical current was first applied to the
cerebral cortex of an anaesthetized dog. Fritsch and Hitzig produced movement in the opposite limbs thus. It seems clear that
the current passed from motor convolution down the cortico-
spinal tract to the contralateral anterior horns of spinal cord and
thus the motor nerves.

This demonstration was followed quickly by the work of Ferrier.
It launched a long series of studies by experimentalists on the
localization of function in the brain. Neurophysiologists entered
the field in brilliant succession: Sherrington to work on reflex
action, Pavlov on conditioned reflexes, Luciani, Graham Brown,
Dusser de Barenne, Vogt, Adrian, Bard, Woolsey, Lashley, Earl
Walker, Bailey, Tower, to name only a few.

Harvey Cushing, American neurosurgeon, first demonstrated
in 1909 that faradic stimulation of the postcentral gyrus of conscious patients produced gross sensation in the opposite limbs.
Other neurosurgeons have since shown that electrical stimulation
of the other primary sensory areas, and the secondary areas as
well, caused patients to see, or hear, or smell, or feel, or taste in an
elementary sort of way.

It has been shown that the rules of facilitation and deviation of
response to electrical stimulation that Sherrington established for
motor responses in the anthropoid cortex apply also to motor and

sensory responses in man (Penfield and Boldrey, 1937; also Penfield and Welch, 1949).

Psychical responses to stimulation, as distinguished from motor or sensory, were produced only more recently. This was stumbled upon quite by accident and was reported in the Harvey Lecture of 1936 (Penfield, 1938). Stimulation in the posterior portion of the right temporal cortex of a patient (J.V.) caused her to re-live an episode of early childhood and to feel fear as she had felt it at the time of the original event. This was an experience that had reappeared to her in dreams also.* In that publication another patient (M.Bu.) was reported who was caused to feel far away, and another was reported who seemed to see herself as she was while giving birth to her child, in the surroundings of that original event.

Such responses to stimulation were reviewed and reported in greater detail in the Ferrier Lecture of 1946 (Penfield, 1947). At that time, ten examples were found, out of 190 cases re-studied, in which stimulation had produced a psychical phenomenon which resembled the "dreamy states" described by Hughlings Jackson.† Jackson was familiar with them during the epileptic fits of patients who had lesions of the temporo-sphenoidal region.

The 190 cases included all craniotomies under local anaesthesia in which stimulation was carried out during a nine year period. The location of stimulations might be anywhere on the accessible cortex. But psychical responses, consisting of *experiential hallucinations* or *interpretive illusions*, were produced only by stimulation of the temporal lobe, as shown in Figure II-11.

Stimulation sometimes caused the patient to have an altered interpretation of the present experience. Everything might seem suddenly familiar or farther away or nearer. These were called perceptual illusions at that time.

In other cases the electrode recalled a previous experience. When point N (Fig. II-11) was stimulated, for example, the patient said, "a familiar sight danced into my mind and away again." The same point was stimulated again, "Yes, three or four things danced

* The case of J.V. has been referred to before. During the past twenty years she has come to be an old friend and is, fortunately, now free of attacks and able to live a happy, constructive life. This was only achieved after eventual removal of the right temporal and occipital lobes in four operations carried out at intervals.

† See Selected Writings of John Hughlings Jackson, 1931, Vol. I.

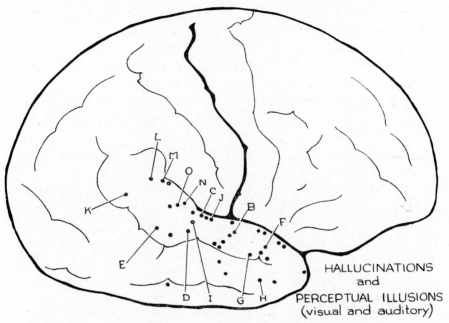

HALLUCINATIONS
and
PERCEPTUAL ILLUSIONS
(visual and auditory)

FIG. II-11. Dots placed on the right hemisphere to summarize the position of points on both sides of the brain where electrical stimulation had produced experiential or interpretive responses during our operations before 1945. All were found to fall on the temporal lobe. From Ferrier Lecture (Penfield, 1946).

before my memory." He was then warned twice falsely and no stimulation was made. Each time he replied, "No."

Stimulation at F caused H.Py. to say, while the stimulation was in progress, "Dream is starting—there are a lot of people in the living room—one of them is my mother."

It is obvious that the mechanism of these psychical responses is of an order very different from that of the motor or sensory responses. The patient recognizes these experiences from his past as authentic. He may have forgotten the event but he does not doubt that it was an experience in which he once played a role. On the other hand, motor and sensory area stimulations are looked upon quite differently.

When the motor convolution is stimulated, the patient may be astonished to discover that he is moving his arm or leg. He may be surprised to hear himself vocalizing, but he never has the impression that he has willed himself to do those things.

When the somatic sensory cortex is stimulated, he reports a sensation of tingling or numbness, or of movement in some particular part. But he is never under the impression that he has touched an external object. He considers it an artifact, not an ordinary sensation.

When the auditory cortex is stimulated, the subject variously describes the sound as ringing, humming, clicking, rushing, chirping, buzzing, knocking, or rumbling. He is never under the impression that he has heard words, nor music, nor anything that represents a memory.

When the visual cortex is stimulated, what the patients see is much more elementary than things seen in ordinary life. They have described what they saw as "flickering lights," "colors," "stars," "wheels," "blue-green and red colored discs," "fawn and blue lights," "colored balls whirling," "radiating gray spots becoming pink and blue," "a long white mark," "shadow moving," "black wheel," etc.

These sensory responses are elementary. An electrode that is delivering, for example, 40, 60, or 80 impulses per second to the "arrival platform" of an area of sensory cortex can hardly be expected to imitate the varied pattern of the stream of impulses that must be arriving normally at that platform when a person sees or feels or hears the things in his environment. Variation in the timing and intensity of potentials, the nerve fibers that are momentarily conducting while other similar fibers are idle, and doubtless other characters, must determine the normal pattern of the afferent stream that reaches the cortical sensory areas. It is this pattern, I suppose, as the stream flows on into the central integrating circuits, that somehow reveals the image of the thing seen or felt or heard.

Cortical conditioning. The presence of frequent abnormal discharges in the region of cortex, which is adjacent to an abnormal area of gray matter that has become epileptogenic, seems to have a conditioning effect. The result of the conditioning is that stimulation from point to point with a gentle electric current reveals evidence of the true function of the cortex with greater ease. Thus the neurosurgeon who explores the cortex with a stimulating electrode may find it easier to map it out functionally if he is not too distant from the focus. For example: The threshold of stimulation may be lower in the motor or sensory area that is near the focus. In the temporal lobe of a patient who has seizures involving that lobe, he may obtain positive responses which would not appear if the epileptogenic discharges were in the frontal lobe.

CHAPTER III

THE RECORDING OF CONSCIOUSNESS AND THE FUNCTION OF INTERPRETIVE CORTEX

W. P.

~~~~~~

~~~~~~

A. *Consciousness*

AT the turn of the 20th century, the psychologist William James wrote these words:

"Consciousness is a personal phenomenon. It deals with external objects, some of which are constant, and it chooses among them. But, in successive moments of time, consciousness is never the same. It is a stream forever flowing, forever changing." (James, 1910).

Heraclitus, the "weeping philosopher" of Ephesus, expressed the thought in fewer words: "We never descend," he said, "twice into the same stream."

In the twenty-four centuries that separated James from Heraclitus, men came to know that the physical basis of consciousness was somehow located in the brain, but they learned little else about the brain. There was almost no advance in knowledge of how man's brain worked. Now, at last, a beginning of understanding is possible, and we should make the most of that beginning.

However, today it is just as difficult to give an adequate definition of the mind as it ever was. Consciousness is an awareness, a thinking, a knowing, a focussing of attention, a planning of action, an interpreting of present experience, a perceiving. These words are descriptive, but they hardly constitute a satisfactory definition.

Fessard (1954) referred to consciousness as the "integrated perception of the present." He was thinking, presumably, of the neuronal mechanism that makes consciousness possible. That is the way a biologist thinks. James, however, was considering primarily its content with no apparent concern for brain mechanisms.

In the awareness of each individual there is a succession of perceptions of the present. The perceptions are made possible by the ever-changing integrative activity of the brain. Perceptions are in one sense separable units since they are held in place for due consideration. But they are not disjointed. They are joined together by the continuous stream of time—the waking time of a man's life-span. They are recorded in the brain in continuity, and yet, separable related experiences are somehow classified and made available for later selective reconsideration. Some of these mechanisms of recall and comparison will be discussed in this chapter, as an introduction to the study of speech.

B. *Psychical responses to stimulation and discharge*

The cerebral cortex is composed of a carpet of nerve cells or ganglion cells that covers the surfaces of the cerebral hemispheres (Fig. III-1). In man this carpet has been vastly increased in extent as compared with the cortex of the brain of other animals. This increase has been made possible by numerous furrows or fissures, so that it has been estimated that only about thirty-five per cent of it lies on the surface. The rest is hidden from sight, dipping inward to form the banks of these fissures.

The human cortex contains many millions of ganglion cells whose insulated axons and dendrites are capable of conducting electrical currents. They are joined together by synaptic junctions, and each area has its fiber connections with ganglionic collections in the centrally placed brain stem. In Chapter II it was pointed out that certain areas of the human cerebral cortex were responsive to electrical stimulation. In this way some areas can be mapped into functional subdivisions and considered as largely sensory or motor (Figs. III-1 and III-2).

The points of positive response that could be called psychical were first collected and summarized in 1946, as shown in Figure II-10. All of them were found to lie on the cortex of one temporal lobe, either right or left. During the eleven years that have elapsed since then, the ability of neurosurgeons to help patients who suffer

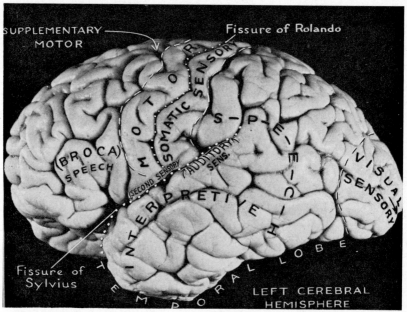

FIG. III-1. Photograph of left hemisphere of the human brain.

from temporal lobe epilepsy has improved, and cases of temporal lobe epilepsy have come to be recognized as constituting the most numerous group among the epilepsies. Consequently, our experience with stimulation in this area of the brain has increased greatly.

The evidence obtained from the responses of conscious patients during the application of an electrode here and there over the cortex must be compared with the evidence derived from study of patients who are subject to spontaneous partial* epileptic discharges in the cortex. In each case there is a localized electrical state in a restricted part of the cortex. This area of cortex is temporarily incapacitated for functional use during the period

* Gastaut (1955) has suggested the word "partial" to describe focal epilepsy in which the electrical disturbance is not generalized.

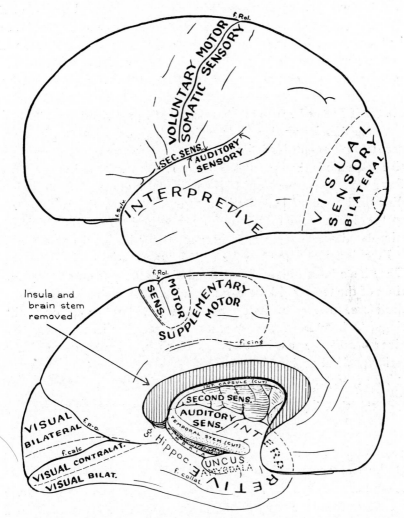

FIG. III-2. Drawing of left hemisphere with sensory, motor, and interpretive areas of cortex labelled roughly. The mesial surface is shown in the lower drawing after the insula has been removed so as to show the deep portion of the superior surface of the temporal lobe and the inferior surfaces of frontal and parietal opercula.

of electrode application. In some areas a positive response may occur as well. In others only silence and localized incapacity results, depending upon the functional nature of the area in question.

Hippocrates used epilepsy as his guide to thinking about the brain. Hughlings Jackson used the evidence presented by epileptic patients as a guide to subdivision of functional areas, although he had uncertain indication as to where the areas might be placed. Jackson was intrigued by discovering "psychical states during the onset of certain epileptic seizures" . . . "dreams mixing up with present thoughts" . . . "double consciousness" . . . "reminiscence" . . . "as if I went back to all that occurred in my childhood."

When the electrical stimulator is applied, or electrical discharge occurs spontaneously, at an epileptogenic focus, and when a positive response is thus produced, there is neuronal conduction away from the area in question. It is conducted by nerve fibers to a less disturbed zone of ganglionic connection. Thus the positive responses identify the function of the ganglionic zone with which the stimulated area has normal, functional cortico-fugal connections.

Psychical responses may be called experiential or interpretive. They have been obtained, as stated above, only from certain portions of the temporal lobe cortex of either hemisphere. It is useful, therefore, to refer to these areas as the *interpretive cortex* to distinguish them from sensory and motor areas and from areas that give no response to stimulation, such as anterior frontal and posterior parietal regions.*

The *interpretive cortex* covers the major portion of each temporal lobe, as suggested by Figure III-2. The left temporal lobe is shown in frontal section in Figures III-3 and III-4. The superior surface of each temporal lobe is hidden within the fissure of Sylvius and circular sulcus. It lies anterior to the auditory sensory cortex of the transverse gyri of Heschl (Fig. III-2, also Fig. II-10). It continues out onto the lateral surface of the temporal lobe, where it extends from the temporal tip backward between the visual and auditory cortex. Whether it covers all of the inferior surface of the temporal lobe is not altogether clear from our evidence at this time, but the mesial surface, including the hippocampal gyrus and uncus, must be considered a part of it.†

The interpretive cortex is continuous, within the depths of

* Complete analysis of the results of stimulation of the human cerebral cortex, as far as our experience goes, may be found in the Sherrington Lecture (Penfield, 1958a). Reference is made to the interpretive cortex in the Proceedings of the National Academy of Sciences (Penfield, 1958b).

† It seems likely that the hippocampus itself plays an indispensable role in the formation or preservation of the actual record of the past, or possibly in its recall.

Sylvian fissure (and beneath that in the circular sulcus), with the gray matter covering the insula, also the deepest extension of the superior opercular banks of fissure and sulcus. Stimulation of

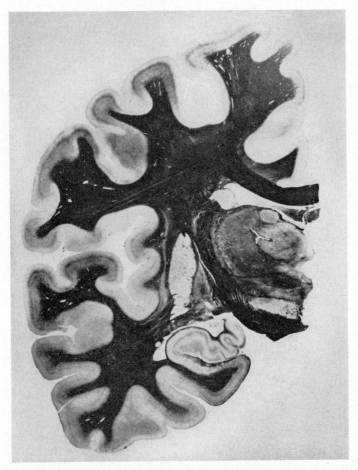

FIG. III-3. Frontal section through left hemisphere to show the extensive infolding of temporal cortex. See surfaces labelled in Fig. III-4. From Jelgersma.*

temporal cortex at this depth sometimes gives rise to responses that one would expect from these neighboring areas: sensation or movement in the alimentary tract suggesting an effect upon the insula, sensations arising in either side of the body such as might

* Jelgersma, G. *Atlas anatomicum cerebri humani.* Scheltema and Holkema, Amsterdam.

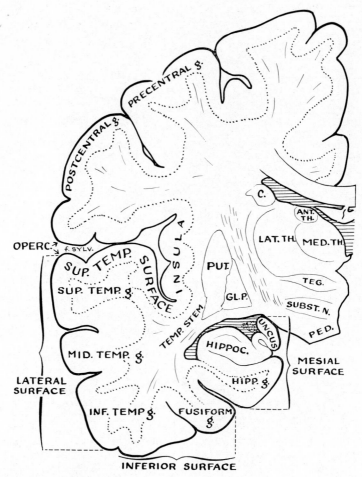

Fɪɢ. III-4. Drawing of frontal section of left hemisphere for comparison with Fig. III-3. From Penfield, 1958c.

be produced from the adjacent second somatic sensory area.* But the psychical responses come only from stimulation of the temporal cortex and occasionally from insular cortex.

It will be pointed out in subsequent chapters that on the

---

* There are also occasional head sensations and abdominal sensations difficult to identify and to locate. Furthermore, when local stimulation produces epileptic discharge in the vicinity of the amygdaloid nucleus, there may be bilateral tonic movement of body and extremities as though there were some closely related motor mechanism there. Epileptic discharge induced by stimulation of the amygdaloid nucleus produces psychomotor confusion, or automatism, during a period for which the patient will later have complete amnesia (Feindel and Penfield, 1954; also Gloor, 1955).

dominant side, the separation between temporal speech cortex and interpretive cortex is not clear. They seem to overlap. But there is no overlapping with the visual sensory cortex of the occipital lobe.

Psychical responses may be divided into two groups: experiential and interpretive.

C. *Experiential responses*

When electrical stimulation recalls the past, the patient has what some of them have called a "flash-back." He seems to re-live some previous period of time and is aware of those things of which he was conscious in that previous period. It is as though the stream of consciousness were flowing again as it did once in the past. Heraclitus said, "We never descend twice into the same stream." But the patient seems to do it. The stream is partially the same but he is aware of something more. He has a double consciousness. He enters the stream of the past and it is the same as it was in the past, but when he looks at the banks of the stream he is aware of the present as well.

During partial epileptic seizures produced by spontaneous discharges in temporal regions, similar phenomena appear. Hughlings Jackson described them and was well aware of the fact that they had to do with the intellect, and that they were more complicated than the sensory and motor manifestations reported by other patients. He called them "dreamy states." Electrical stimulation produces these same "states" and usually does so without producing a seizure or epileptic after-discharge.

Take as an example the words of M.Ma. during stimulation of her right temporal lobe. The brain had been exposed as suggested in Figure III-5. When an electrode, insulated except at the tip, was introduced through point 17 (Fig. III-5) one centimeter into the cortex of the superior surface of the temporal lobe and a gentle current was switched on, she exclaimed:

"Oh, a familiar memory—in an office somewhere. I could see the desks. I was there and someone was calling to me—a man leaning on a desk with a pencil in his hand."

All the detail of those things to which she had paid attention in some previous period of time were still there. Perhaps the pencil

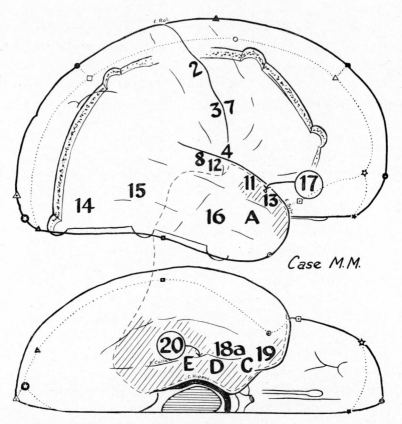

FIG. III-5. CASE M.Ma. at operation. Extent of exposure of right hemisphere is indicated by sketch of skull edge. Some positive responses to the stimulations carried out are indicated by the numbers. Letters E, D, and C indicate site of epileptogenic discharge detected by electro-corticography. Shaded areas indicate abnormality; broken line, the extent of surgical removal of the temporal lobe which has resulted in cessation of seizures during the 5 years since operation. From Penfield, 1954b.

in his hand had seemed important, but other images that must have reached her retina during the original experience are now lost, probably because they were ignored originally.

After removal of the superior and lateral portions of the temporal lobe as far back as the broken line (Fig. III-5), leaving the mesial portion of the lobe intact, stimulation at point 18a caused her to say:

"I had a little memory—a scene from a play. They were talking and I could see it. It was just seeing it in my memory."

It was possible also to place the electrode at point 20 (Fig. III-5) on the lateral surface of the hippocampal gyrus, since the adjacent fusiform gyrus had been removed (compare "hip. G" and "fusiform G," Fig. III-4). This caused her to say:

"A familiar memory—the place where I hang my coat up—where I go to work."

When this stimulation of hippocampal gyrus was carried out, the hippocampal formation and amygdaloid nucleus were still intact. But the rest of the anterior half of the temporal lobe had been removed. The fact that stimulation (at 20 and 18a) could still produce a flash-back of former experience would support the suggestion that comes from other evidence (Milner and Penfield, 1958) that the hippocampus of the two sides is, in fact, the repository of ganglionic patterns that preserve the record of the stream of consciousness. If not the repository, then each hippocampus plays an important role in the mechanism of re-activation of that record.

D. *Interpretive responses*

These responses are interpretations of the present, of which the patient becomes suddenly aware. We may refer again to patient M.Ma. When the electrode was applied to point 14, also 15, it produced a sudden sense of familiarity which she referred at once to her present experience. She felt that the operation had happened before and that she even knew what the surgeon was about to do. This occurred without any recall of the past. It was a subconscious conclusion. Under normal circumstances such conclusions are based on actual experience from the past.

When such interpretations have been described by patients afflicted with temporal lobe epilepsy, clinicians have long called them "déjà vu" (already seen) phenomena. They are false interpretations of the present and therefore are called illusions. But these illusions take other forms as well. There may be a false sense of familiarity as already described. Or, on the contrary, everything may seem strange or absurd. The relationship of the individual to his environment may seem to be altered. The distance from things seen or heard may seem to be increased or decreased. The patient may say that he feels far away from himself or from the world.

47

Allied to these altered interpretations is the production of emotions not justified by the present experience. Fear is the commonest emotion produced by stimulation. It was reported, as an epileptic aura, 22 times out of 271 cases of temporal lobe epilepsy analyzed by Mullan and Penfield (1959), and was produced by stimulation 9 times during operation on such patients.

All of these are interpretive responses. They correspond with the useful judgments which a normal individual is making constantly as he compares present experience with past experience. If a decision is to be made as to whether present experience is familiar, or appropriate, or menacing, the record of past experience must be available, and the new record must be somehow classified and compared with similar old records for the purpose of comparison.

However, under normal circumstances these signals of interpretation rise into consciousness suddenly, as the result of subconscious comparative interpretation. There is little or no voluntary effort to recall previous similar experience for the purpose of comparison.

E. *Location of interpretive cortex*

Both types of response, experiential and interpretive, argue for the existence of a permanent ganglionic recording of the stream of consciousness. The record of that stream must be preserved in a specialized mechanism. Otherwise, experiential responses to an electrode applied locally would be impossible. It seems likely also that appropriate parts of this same record are somehow utilized when recurring judgments are made in regard to familiarity and the meaning of each new experience.

These psychical responses, as already pointed out, were produced by stimulation of the temporal cortex (Fig. III-2), chiefly on the superior and lateral surfaces of both lobes and probably extending a little way into the parietal lobe. They were also produced by stimulation of the remaining hippocampal gyrus after removal of most of the rest of the temporal lobe.

No psychical responses resulted from stimulation of other lobes. It seems fair to conclude, therefore, that these areas of cortex have a particular relationship to the *record of experience* and the reactivation of that record.

F. *Discussion*

One might assume that during his normal life, a man makes employment of the interpretive cortex under the following circumstances:

Mr. A. meets Mr. B. unexpectedly. He is aware of a sudden signal, or feeling, of familiarity. "A" must, therefore, have made an instantaneous comparison of "B" as he enters his field of vision, with the old records of "B" from past experiences. He does this in a subconscious process. More than that, he seems to have acquired a clearer picture of the former "B" than he had a moment earlier, for he is able now to detect trifling changes in the appearance or the movement or voice of his friend.

One may conclude that if, during a surgical operation, such signals of present interpretation result from temporal cortex stimulation, and if, at other times, the flash-back record of the past is unlocked by stimulation there, the temporal cortex normally plays a role in the interpretation of present experience. It might be assumed further that this cortex has a mechanism for scanning and selection of similar experiences from the past record.

Before Mr. A, in the foregoing parable, can name his friend, he must employ another partly separable mechanism, the *speech mechanism*. To do this, he must make use of other areas of cortex which serve the specialized purposes of finding the name he has formerly associated with this person.

The *interpretive cortex* is that portion of the cerebral cortex in which electrical stimulation may elicit experiential and interpretive responses to stimulation.

In order to produce an *experiential response*, a ganglionic record must be activated. But we should not necessarily conclude that the record mechanism is actually in the gray matter where the electrode is being applied. On the contrary, one might expect that the local effect of electricity, within a considerable distance surrounding the point of application, would prevent the activation of any elaborate and complicated local mechanism. But a stream of neuronal impulses might well leave the area of electrical application and be conducted along nerve fibers to some more distant area where the ganglionic record could thus be activated in a normal physiological manner.

49

That is actually the situation in regard to the motor gyrus, as was pointed out in Chapter II. No delicate or elaborate movements of hand or foot can be evoked by electrical stimulation of the cortex. The only elaborate responses obtained are those of vocalization, swallowing, conjugate looking movements of the eyes; and it seems clear that these are all produced by conduction from the precentral gyrus along nerve fiber connections to more distant neuronal mechanisms in the brain stem—mechanisms that are available to the motor cortex of both hemispheres (Penfield, 1958a).

Thus the actual record of the stream of consciousness may well be in the hippocampus of both sides—a possibility that is strongly supported by the results of bilateral injury to, or removal of, the hippocampal zone (Milner and Penfield, 1955)—or it might be in some deeper structure.

On the other hand, the so called *interpretive responses*, which are, in a sense, simple and similar from case to case (judgments of familiarity, strangeness, distance, intensity, loneliness, fear), might well result from local cortical activity near the electrode, conducting to undetermined subcortical targets.

1. *The patient's view of these phenomena*

When stimulation has produced an experiential response during operative exploration, the patient has usually recognized that this was something out of his own past. At the same time he may have been acutely aware of the fact that he was lying upon the operating table. Thus, he was able to contemplate and to talk about this doubling of awareness and to recognize it as a strange paradox.

A young man, J.T. (Penfield and Jasper, 1954, p. 136), who had recently come from his home in South Africa, cried out when the superior surface of his right temporal lobe was being stimulated: "Yes, Doctor! Yes, Doctor! Now I hear people laughing—my friends—in South Africa." After stimulation was over, he could discuss his double awareness and express his astonishment, for it had seemed to him that he was with his cousins at their home where he and the two young ladies were laughing together. He did not remember what they were laughing at. Doubtless he would have discovered that also, if the strip of experience had begun earlier, or if the surgeon had continued the stimulation a little longer.

This was an experience from his earlier life. It had faded from his recollective memory, but the ganglionic pattern which must have been formed during that experience was still intact and available to the stimulating electrode. It was at least as clear to him as it would have been had he closed his eyes and ears thirty seconds after the event and rehearsed the whole scene "from memory." Sight and sound and personal interpretation—all were re-created for him by the electrode.

It is significant, however, that during the re-creation of that past experience he was not impelled to speak to his cousins. Instead, he spoke to the "Doctor" in the operating room. Herein may lie an important distinction between this form of hallucination and the hallucinations of a patient during a toxic delirium or a psychotic state. In my experience (and relying only on my own memory, which is far from perfect!) no patient has ever addressed himself to a person who was part of a past experience, unless perhaps it was when he had passed into a state of automatism.*

2. Flash-back of experience contrasted with recollective memory

Some patients call an experiential response a dream. Others state that it is a "flash-back" from their own life history. All agree that it is more vivid than anything that they could recollect voluntarily.

G.F. (Penfield and Jasper, 1954, p. 137) was caused to hear her small son, Frank, speaking in the yard outside her own kitchen, and she heard the "neighborhood sounds" as well. Ten days after the operation she was asked if this was a memory. "Oh, no," she replied. "It seemed more real than that." Then she added, "Of course, I have heard Frankie like that many, many times—thousands of times."

This response to stimulation was a single experience. Her memory of such occasions was a generalization. Without the aid of the electrode she could not recall any one of the specific instances nor hear the honking of automobiles that might mean danger to Frankie, or cries of other children or the barking of

* During automatism patients sometimes talk about unrelated matters, which might suggest that they were addressing someone, but after it is over they never describe hallucinations and there is complete subsequent amnesia.

dogs that would have made up the "neighborhood sounds" on each occasion.

The patients have never looked upon an experiential response as a remembering. Instead of that it is a hearing-again and seeing-again—a living-through moments of past time.

D.F. listened to an orchestra in the operating room but did not recall where she had heard it "that way." It was a song she had never learned to sing or play. Perhaps she had been oblivious of her surroundings while she listened to the orchestra in that previous period of time. T.S. heard music and seemed to be in the theatre where he had heard it. A.Bra. heard the singing of a Christmas song in her church at home in Holland. She seemed to be there in the church and was moved again by the beauty of the occasion, just as she had been on that Christmas Eve some years before.*

The experience goes forward. There are no still pictures. The flash-back has strong visual and auditory components, but always it is an unfolding of sight and sound and also, though rarely, of sense of position. Curiously enough, no patient has yet reported pain or taste or smell during an experiential response, although they have been produced as simple sensory phenomena. It should be said, however, that the failure to get a response of any particular type has little statistical value, for the total number of patients from whom psychical responses have been elicited is, after all, small.†

It is clear that each successive recording is somehow classified and compared with previous recordings so that, little by little, each separate song is "learned" and becomes a unit in memory. And all the familiar things in a man's life undergo the same change. A poem or an elocution may be "committed to memory." But *memory*, as we ordinarily think of it, is something more, and a great deal less than any recording, unless that recording was made unusually vivid by fear or joy or special meaning. Then perhaps the detail of an original experience and the patient's memory of it might be identical. In that case memory and flash-back would be the same.

* More complete descriptions of all these cases and others may be found by initials in the Case Index. See Penfield and Jasper, 1954.

† The positive responses are acceptable as facts, for they were carefully checked in every instance. But little weight should be placed on what is not observed.

DISCUSSION

The experiential responses of the flash-back variety were, for the most part, quite unimportant moments in the patient's life; standing on a street corner, hearing a mother call her child, taking part in a conversation, listening to a little boy as he played in the yard. If these unimportant minutes of time were preserved in the ganglionic recordings of these patients, why should it be thought that any experience in the stream of consciousness drops out of the ganglionic record.

When, by chance, the neurosurgeon's electrode activates past experience, that experience unfolds progressively, moment by moment. This is a little like the performance of a wire recorder or a strip of cinematographic film on which are registered all those things of which the individual was once aware—the things he selected for his attention in that interval of time. Absent from it are the sensations he ignored, the talk he did not heed.

Time's strip of film runs forward, never backward, even when resurrected from the past. It seems to proceed again at time's own unchanged pace. It would seem, once one section of the strip has come alive, that the response is protected by a functional all-or-nothing principle. A regulating inhibitory mechanism must guard against activation of other portions of the film. As long as the electrode is held in place, the experience of a former day goes forward. There is no holding it still, no turning back, no crossing with other periods. When the electrode is withdrawn, it stops as suddenly as it began.

A particular strip can sometimes be repeated by interrupting the stimulation and then shortly reapplying it at the same or a nearby point. In that case it begins at the same moment of time on each occasion. The threshold of evocation of that particular response has apparently been lowered for a time by the first stimulus. Graham Brown and Sherrington (1912) described local facilitation and intensification of motor responses by repeated stimulation at a single point in the anthropoid cortex, and we have found the same to be true for man in motor and sensory areas of the cortex (Penfield and Rasmussen, 1950).

Similar rules of facilitation seem to be applicable to the interpretive cortex as well. And here the effect of one stimulation upon the response to subsequent stimulations, at the same or different points, seems to be far greater and longer lasting.

53

Eccles (1951) has suggested that: "Memory of all events is dependent on the development and persistence of increased excitatory efficacy across certain synaptic junctions." He supported his argument by pointing out that he and McIntyre had demonstrated that "activation of monosynaptic paths in the spinal cord led to prolonged (measured in hours and possibly days) increase in the excitatory efficacy of synaptic knobs rendered specially sensitive by disuse."

The existence of the flash-back responses indicates that nerve cells and junctions employed in the preservation of the record retain "increased excitatory efficacy" for a far longer period—most of an individual's lifetime, in fact.

G. *Conclusion*

Every individual forms a neuronal record of his own stream of consciousness. Since artificial re-activation of the record, later in life, seems to re-create all those things formerly included within the focus of his attention, one must assume that the re-activated recording and the original neuronal activity are identical. Thus, the recorded pattern of neuronal activity may be considered much more than a record, for it was once used as the final stage of integration to make consciousness what it was. One might suppose that originally, like a strip of film, its meaning was projected on the screen of man's awareness, and somehow it was held in place there for a brief time of consideration before it was replaced by subsequent experience and subsequent neuronal patternings.

Consciousness, "forever flowing" past us, makes no record of itself, and yet the recording of its counterpart within the brain is astonishingly complete. This counterpart, made up of the passing of potentials through the everchanging circuits of final integration, is recorded in temporal succession between the experience which went before and that which follows.

The thread of time remains with us in the form of a succession of "abiding" facilitations. This thread travels through ganglion cells and synaptic junctions. It runs through the waking hours of each man, from childhood to the grave. On the thread of time are strung, like pearls in unending succession, the "meaningful" pat-

terns that can still recall the vanished content of a former awareness.*

No man can voluntarily reactivate the record. Perhaps, if he
could, he might become hopelessly confused. Man's voluntary
recollection must be achieved through other mechanisms. And yet
the recorded patterns are useful to him, even after the passage of
many years. They can still be appropriately selected by some scanning process and activated with amazing promptness for the purposes of comparative interpretation. It is, it seems to me, in this
mechanism of recall and comparison and interpretation that the
interpretive cortex of the temporal lobes plays its specialized role.

* The words "abiding" and "meaningful" in this paragraph are taken from
Sherrington's oft-quoted (Adrian, 1947, p. 17) description of the fully awakened
brain as "an enchanted loom where millions of flashing shuttles weave a dissolving
pattern, always a meaningful pattern though never an abiding one."

CHAPTER IV

ANALYSIS OF LITERATURE

L. R.

〜〜〜〜〜〜〜〜〜〜〜〜〜〜〜〜〜〜〜〜〜〜〜〜〜〜〜〜

A. On aphasia
B. On agnosia and apraxia
C. On localization

〜〜〜〜〜〜〜〜〜〜〜〜〜〜〜〜〜〜〜〜〜〜〜〜〜〜〜〜

A. *On aphasia*

IN 1861 there was a considerable argument between those who believed that the cerebral hemispheres function as a whole and those who contended that there is localization of function in the cerebrum. *Gall* (Gall and Spurzheim, 1810-1819) had performed excellent work on the anatomy of the brain but was criticized for his unscientific system of phrenology. *Bouillaud* (1825) maintained, on the basis of examination of brains of patients who had had loss of speech, that the cerebral control of movements necessary for speech resided in the frontal lobes, and he thus supported Gall. Against the teachings of *Flourens* (1824) that all parts of the cerebrum were equipotential, Bouillaud pointed out that paresis of one part of the body as the result of a cerebral lesion could not occur were this true.

Marc Dax had read a paper in Montpellier in 1836, stating that loss of speech was associated with right hemiplegia and therefore due to a lesion on the left hemisphere. However, this was unknown in Paris, as the paper was not presented by Dax's son until 1863 and was not published until 1865. It should be emphasized that the discovery of the motor area in animals by Fritsch and Hitzig was not until 1870, and, indeed, the observations of *Broca* probably furnished the incentive for this experiment.

Paul Broca (Fig. IV-1) was secretary of the Société d'Anthropologie in 1861, at a time when these heated discussions were occurring. He was a surgeon and a good anatomist. He believed in the principle of localization, chiefly based on the embryological and anatomical work of Gall, Gratiolet, and himself.

Broca had a patient, Leborgne, who was to serve as a test case.

This 51-year-old man had had seizures since his youth. At the age of 30 he lost his speech (the circumstances of which were unknown) and was admitted to Bicêtre. He was only able to say "tan" and to curse, "Sacré nom de D. . . ." His companions detested him and even called him a thief. At the age of 40 he gradually developed paralysis of the right arm and leg, and by the age of

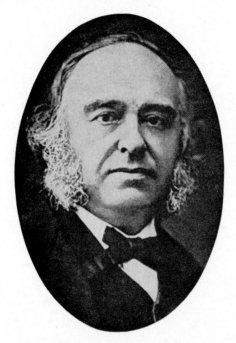

FIG. IV-1. Photograph of Pierre Paul Broca (1824-1880). He was a noted French surgeon who first described aphemia as due to a lesion of the posterior part of the third frontal convolution.

44, became bedridden. Over the patient's last ten years he had increasing difficulty in vision. His sheets were changed once a week, and it was discovered that he had a diffuse cellulitis of the right leg, for which he was transferred to the service of Broca.

On examination he had no movement of the right arm and leg. His left cheek was blown out more than the right on whistling.* He had difficulty in swallowing. There was decreased sensation to pain over the right side. He could not write. He was able to indi-

* Broca believed that there was weakness of the ipsilateral face and contralateral extremities with lesions of the cerebral hemispheres.

cate the length of time he had been in Bicêtre, could tell the time, and gave the order of appearance of his difficulties (pointed to mouth, then to right arm and leg). Some of the things a normal person could have indicated by pantomime, he could not. His only speech was "tan" and swearing. He died shortly afterwards.

The brain weighed 987 grams. The orbital and first frontal convolutions were atrophic, but there was no break in the surface of the cortex. A cystic cavity occupied the posterior part of the third frontal with the adjacent part of the second frontal and precentral convolutions. The ascending parietal, angular, first temporal, and part of second temporal gyri, and the insula were also involved. Through a hole into the ventricle, accidently made by Broca, the corpus striatum was seen to be softened.

The second patient of Broca was an 84-year-old man named Lelong. He was transferred to Broca's service because of a fracture of the left femur. Nine and a half years before, he had had loss of consciousness, from which he recovered in a few days without paralysis but with "aphémie." He was admitted to Bicêtre eighteen months later with senile debility, feebleness, tremor, and inability to work or to write. His sight, hearing, motor power (except in fractured extremity), and sensation were stated to be normal. His only words were "Oui, non, tois (trois), toujour, and Lelo (Lelong)." When asked if he knew how to write, he replied, "Oui;" if he could write, "Non." When he tried, he was unable to manage the pen. He indicated that he had been in hospital eight years, that he had two sons and two daughters, that he was eighty-four years old, and that it was ten o'clock; but he always used the word "tois." He made gestures of digging and planting to indicate his former occupation.

Lelong died twelve days after the fracture. His brain weighed 1,136 grams. There was a collection of fluid about the size of a franc over the posterior end of the third frontal convolution, and loss of substance extended over fifteen millimeters. The cortex of the second frontal convolution was only two millimeters thick. There was a separate lesion of softening at the junction of the anterior end of the corpus striatum with the white matter of the frontal lobe.

On the basis of these two cases, Broca contended that the center for articulate speech was the posterior part of the third frontal convolution. He stated that whether it were anterior or whether it were posterior in the frontal lobe might not be important, but that it was the third convolution. *Pierre Marie* (1926) has criticized these two cases by implying that Broca did not give full anatomical descriptions of the surface lesions in the first case, and that there was only the expected appearance of senility in the second. Neither of these criticisms is valid. The three most important criticisms are: 1) there is no proof of Broca's supposition that the lesion of the third frontal convolution was the oldest in the first case; 2) examination of the patients was inadequate according to present-day standards; and 3) neither brain has been sectioned, so that any anatomical conclusion is unjustifiable.

At any rate, these cases caused almost everyone interested in neurology to participate in the reporting of new material and to discuss cerebral localization. According to *Broca* (1888), Charcot reported the next three cases, and Gubler another, of disease of the third frontal convolutions with *aphemia*. Charcot and then Trousseau found lesions of the parietal lobe with aphemia, but Broca discovered a lesion of the third frontal gyrus in each. Then Charcot reported two more lesions of the third frontal convolution with speech disturbance. The preceding ten cases all involved the left hemisphere. Levy had a patient with a lesion of the same area on the right side without speech disturbance, and Charcot reported *aphemia* with a lesion of the left parietal lobe, to which Broca agreed.

Broca stated that the *fundamentals of speech* consist of 1) an idea; 2) connection which convention had established between idea and word; 3) the art of combining movements of organs of articulation with the suitable words; and 4) the use of the organs of articulation. Loss of ideas was termed *"alogie."* Loss of conventional connections between idea and word was *"amnésie verbale"* of Lordat. Patients with this disorder used words which had no connection with the idea; they had forgotten the special memory of spoken and written words; but they still had memory as they recognized objects, places, and persons. Loss of the art of combining movements of organs of articulation with the suitable words was *"aphémie."* These patients might have no words, few words (particularly curse words), strange words in no vocabulary, or a more extended vocabulary. Distinction between this patient and the previous one was that the aphemic patient understood what was said to him. Damage to muscle, nerve, or brain controlling nerve was *"alalie mécanique."*

Broca criticized Trousseau's substitution of "aphasie" for "aphémie," in that "aphasie" meant without phases of the moon or brightness, or without ideas (Plato). According to Trousseau, the Greek meaning of "aphémie" in 1861 was infamy! Broca later suggested that the indefinite term "aphasie" be used for indefinite cases, as M. Trousseau had used it with his inexact descriptions; and if the case be classifiable, it would be one of the four preceding. However, Broca admitted that he had diagnosed "amnésie verbale" and found a lesion in the same place as for "aphémie."

Following the French school, the English and Germans took up the study of aphasia (the term which had come into general use). In 1867, *Ogle* published a case of a man who could write things that he could not say, suggested that writing was separate from speech, and introduced the term *agraphia* to apply to patients who were unable to write.

Bastian began writing on aphasia in 1869 and continued for some thirty years. He was the first to describe *"word-deafness"* and *"word-blindness."* The former was supposed to be a condition in which the patient had no difficulty hearing but was unable to recognize a word as such, and the latter was a similar condition in which the patient was able to see normally but could not recognize a word. Bastian believed that one thought in words, and that there were different specific centers with fiber connections: auditory and visual word centers, "glosso-" and "cheiro-kinesthesic" centers. He stated that destruction of Broca's area produced loss of kinesthetic memory. He traced the development of speech in the child, just as Broca had done, and believed the auditory word center to be the most important.

Wernicke (1874) published a monograph of seventy-two pages in a great part of which he emphasized the work of Meynert in tracing sensory pathways, particularly visual, to the cortex, and the experiments of Fritsch and Hitzig. He believed that the anterior half of the brain was concerned with the concept of movement and the posterior (including the temporal lobe) with sensory impressions; the cells of the cortex were, he thought, neither motor nor sensory but depended on their connections to determine their function.

Wernicke separated the general auditory area from the *auditory speech area* and located the latter in the first temporal convolution. A lesion in the auditory speech area would produce loss of understanding of speech. There would be difficulty in naming and in speaking, as one could not understand in order to correct the mistakes. In addition, the patient would have inability to read and to write, due to the learning process of hearing words while reading and writing (though an educated person might be able to read silently, though not aloud). He stated that there were various degrees of difficulty in understanding; there might be loss of "Klangbilder" or just loss of "Bindewörter" for sentence formation. He drew diagrams with the centers located: auditory speech in first temporal; Broca's motor speech area, third frontal; and writing, second frontal gyrus (Fig. IV-2).

Wernicke proceeded to give ten cases, only three of which had autopsies, and two of these showed diffuse lesions. One case had a lesion of the posterior part of the first temporal and adjacent second temporal convolutions. He was satisfied that there was an auditory word center and that it was located in the first temporal convolution.

Kussmaul (1877) desired to make word-deafness and word-blindness separate entities. He accepted the work of *Finkelnburg* (1870), who pointed out that patients with cerebral lesions might have disorders not directly connected with word formation: "*asymboly*" was the inability to express ideas by means of signs, together with lack of understanding of their significance. Kussmaul believed that speech could not be located in one or another particular convolution. Nonetheless, he proceeded with a very complicated diagram. This diagram was not received as well as that of Broadbent (1878), with its naming and propositionizing centers as well as visual, tactile, auditory, and speech centers; or that of Lichtheim (1885), with its visual, auditory, writing, motor, and multiple concept centers. The cases, however, could not be fitted into any of these schemata.

Hughlings Jackson (1931) (Fig. IV-3) stated that speech was a psychical act, and warned against classifications which were partly anatomical and physiological and partly psychological. "These mixed classifications lead to the use of such expressions as that an *idea* of a word produces an articulatory *movement*: whereas a psychical state, an 'idea of a word' (or simply 'a word'), cannot produce an articulatory movement, a physical state." (p. 156)

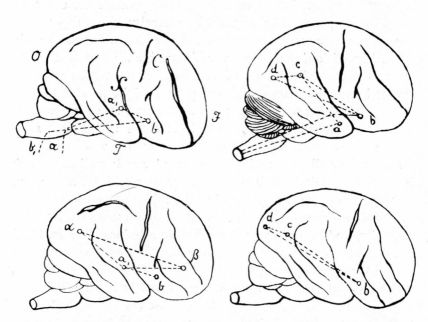

FIG. IV-2. Wernicke's drawings (1874) to show his belief in speech localization. The upper left drawing shows the auditory center a,, and Broca's area b. The upper right picture shows c as being the a,, plus the associated picture which is formed by obtaining a visual picture through touch; and d is the optic memory picture center. In the lower left drawing alpha is the center for the visual memory picture of the letter, and beta is the writing center in the second frontal convolution. In the lower right drawing c and d represent centers for tactile and visual letters, the exact locus being unknown but not in the first temporal convolution. The broken lines indicate Wernicke's surmise as to conduction pathways.

"To coin the word, verbalising, to include all ways in which words serve, I would assert that both halves of the brain are alike in that each serves in *verbalising*. That the left half does is evident, because damage of it makes a man speechless. That the right does is inferable, because the speechless man understands all I say to him in ordinary matters." (p. 132)

"When we consider more fully the duality of the verbalising process, of which the second 'half' is speech, we shall try to show that there is a duality also in the revival of the images symbolised; that perception is the termination of a stage beginning by the unconscious or subconscious revival of images which are in effect 'image-symbols'; that we think not only by aid of those symbols,

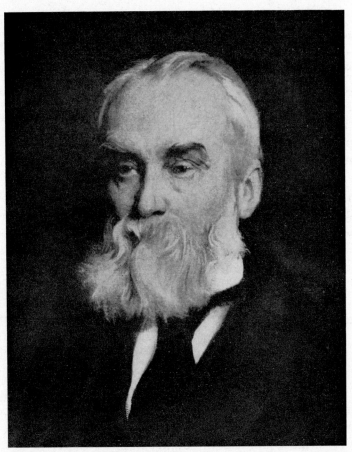

Fig. IV-3. Photograph of John Hughlings Jackson (1835-1911). He was one of the leading neurologists of his time and contributed much to the understanding of speech mechanisms.

ordinarily so-called (words), but by aid of symbol-images. It is, I think, because speech and perception are preceded by an unconscious or subconscious reproduction of words and images, that we seem to have 'faculties' of speech and of perception, as it were, above and independent of the rest of ourselves." (pp. 167-168)

"I think that the left is the side for the automatic revival of images and the right the side for their voluntary revival—for recognition" (p. 142). "Thus, very sudden and very extensive damage to *any part* of the left cerebral hemisphere would produce *some* amount of defect of speech, and I believe that similar damage to any part of the right hemisphere might produce *some* defect of recognition." (p. 142)

Jackson believed that the destruction of Broca's area produced aphasia, but he did not localize speech in any particular part. He thought the nervous arrangements of Broca's region represented movements of tongue, palate, lips, larynx, and pharynx.

He stressed the fact that the aphasic has lost propositional speech but may have emotional speech, recurrent utterances, and, rarely, propositions. He believed that these are mediated through the right hemisphere as well as "jargon," which is the survival of the fittest under the circumstances. Again, Jackson stated that a lesion does not produce positive symptoms, but that the activity of a lower level released from control of the higher level gives the positive effects. The negative condition consists of inability to speak, to write (he is able to copy and frequently to sign his name), to read; and the ability to pantomime is defective. The patient's positive symptoms are ability to understand what is said or read to him, to move his articulatory organs well in eating, drinking and in such utterances as remain possible, to use his vocal organs, and to use emotional language.

Jackson described the first case of partial imperception in a patient who at times did not recognize objects, persons, or places, and who put her clothes on backwards. She had several tumors in the right temporo-occipital region.

Jackson (1868) reported the first case of a left-handed man with a lesion of the right hemisphere and aphasia; however, he probably did not know it was the first case, as he seemed to have accepted the theory that aphasia would accompany disease of the right hemisphere in the left-handed.

Jackson's contributions to the understanding of aphasia are great, even though some of his and Spencer's (1892) psychological theories are not acceptable today.

In 1873, *Ferrier* (1886) localized the *auditory center* in animals in the temporal lobe. *Munk* (1877) determined the visual cortex to be in the occipital region of animals and demonstrated "*mind-*

*blindness."** These animal experiments had profound effects upon clinical interpretations.

In 1881, *Dejerine* (1914) stated that word-blindness was due to a lesion of the angular gyrus, and he later maintained that a lesion of the angular gyrus produced word-blindness, total agraphia, and paraphasia. At the same time *Exner* maintained that the second frontal gyrus is the writing center, in agreement with Wernicke. *Mills* (1895) placed a naming center in the third temporal convolution. All of these contentions were based on totally inadequate materials.

The interest in aphasia decreased at the beginning of this century—probably because of the difficulty of fitting the individual case to the various schemata—until *Pierre Marie* (1906) wrote: "La troisième circonvolution frontal gauche ne joue aucun rôle spécial dans la fonction du langage."†

Marie's basic criticisms were that the anatomical material was not adequate to allow the conclusions drawn, and that the clinical testing of the patients had been insufficient. He maintained that all aphasics have some defect in comprehension; they may be able to respond adequately to simple questions but fail on the more complicated ones (e.g. Marie's "test of three papers"). In addition, he stated that general intelligence is lowered; the patient is by no means demented, but he is unable to do some things not directly related to speech, for example: solving simple arithmetic problems or cooking an egg by a "chef." He correctly emphasized the fact that the patients Broca reported were not able to understand everything and were unable to write (ability to read was not stated in Broca's first two accounts).

Marie maintained that *Wernicke's aphasia* was the true aphasia; the patient comprehends speech insufficiently, speaks poorly with paraphasia and jargon, is unable to read and to write, and presents a particular intellectual deficit. He defined anarthria as not only a difficulty in articulation due to a disturbance in movement of the anatomical parts concerned in speech, but also a loss of control of those acts directly necessary for the production of speech; he

---

* As Lashley (1948) pointed out, Loeb denied the interpretation that vision was intact in Munk's animals and considered the visual field to be narrowed; this was confirmed by the experiments of Hitzig.

† "The left third frontal convolution does not play any special role in the function of language."

stated that it was equivalent to the subcortical motor aphasia of Pitres and was due to a lesion of the "lenticular zone" of either hemisphere (Fig. IV-4). Broca's aphasia was therefore Wernicke's aphasia plus anarthria.

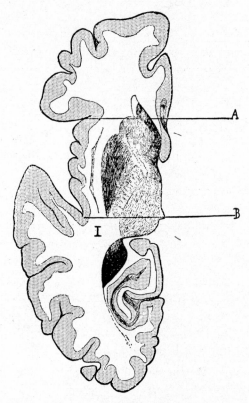

FIG. IV-4. Photograph of Pierre Marie's lenticular zone. He stated that involvement of this zone in either hemisphere produced motor disturbance in speech, whereas involvement of Wernicke's zone of the dominant hemisphere produced "true aphasia."

Marie was able to present a case of a right-handed man who was blind from glaucoma and was violent and demented, but who presented no difficulty in speech; the lesion, as seen at autopsy, destroyed the posterior part of the third frontal convolution. However, the precentral gyrus was not identified microscopically in this case.

In the "Discussion sur l'aphasie" at the meetings of the Neurological Society of Paris (1908) Madame Dejerine showed that the lenticular zone of Marie contained fibers from Broca's area. The discussions centered around Marie's concept of anarthria and the function of the third frontal convolution; and they failed to emphasize his more important criticisms as regards the nature of aphasia, and his contention that the pure psychical images necessary for speech cannot be localized.

Monakow (1897-1914) introduced the concept of *diaschisis* to explain the temporary effects of a cerebral lesion. This constitutes the lowering or abolition of activity of those cells in uninjured areas which are in direct anatomical and physiological connection with the local area of injury. This is not the generalized effect of shock but a specific localized condition. In recovery the effects of shock and edema first pass off, then those of diaschisis (over a period of weeks or months); the oldest, most organized activities return before the more complex. With this concept *Monakow* localized areas the destruction of which produced definite clinical syndromes, but he insisted that there were no centers.

Henschen (1920-1922) became the foremost proponent of cerebral localization. He reviewed the literature on aphasia which consisted of about 1350 cases. He deplored the lack of clinical and anatomical data but, nonetheless, drew the most extravagant conclusions from these same cases. His contribution was great, though, in making available the summaries of all these cases.

Pick (1913) and *Head* (1926) emphasized the importance of Hughlings Jackson's contributions to the study of aphasia. Head maintained that a cerebral lesion produces more than a disorder of speech (in those cases where speech is affected), and he said, "symbolic formulation and expression" suffer in these cases. He insisted that the word is not the unit of speech. "Not only is it impossible to break up a word into auditory and visual elements, but disease does not analyze a sentence into its verbal or grammatical constituents. We cannot assume that a sentence is strictly a unit of speech. Speech, like walking, is an act of progression." (Vol. 1, p. 120)

Head divided aphasia into four groups: verbal, syntactical, nominal, and semantic. The most original of these was the semantic aphasia, which he defined as follows: "These defects are characterised by lack of recognition of the full significance of words and phrases apart from their immediate verbal meaning. The patient

67

fails to comprehend the final aim or goal of an action initiated spontaneously or imposed upon him from without. He cannot formulate accurately, either to himself or to others, a general conception of what he has been told, has read to himself, or has seen in a picture, although he is able to enumerate most of the details. Such patients understand what is said, can read and can write, but the result tends to be inaccurate and confused. Counting is possible and the relative value of coins may be recognized, but arithmetical operations are affected and the patient is commonly confused by the monetary transactions of daily life. Drawing even from a model is usually defective and in most instances construction of a simple ground-plan is impossible. Orientation is definitely disturbed. The patient finds considerable difficulty in laying the table, putting together portions of some object he has constructed, or in planning an operation he desires to perform. This interferes seriously with his activities in daily life and renders him useless for any but the simplest employment; and yet his memory and intelligence may remain on a comparatively high general level." (Vol. 2, pp. xix and xx)

Head found these various disturbances in several patients, but they may occur separately. Perhaps they are disturbances in "symbolic formulation and expression." However, usually they are not considered as a type of aphasia. As he pointed out, they may occur with damage of the right hemisphere.

Head's work would have been more valuable if he had not felt it necessary to indicate the site of the lesion which would give the different types of aphasia he described (Fig. IV-5). He based this classification on only eleven cases. All were gunshot or shrapnel wounds except one—a compound skull fracture from the kick of a horse. The accuracy of the localization without the benefit of autopsy or cortical stimulation is extremely doubtful. Subsequent authors have not agreed with this classification.

Marie and *Foix* (1917) summarized their study of aphasia from war wounds. Lesions in the region of zone A (Fig. IV-6) produce anarthria. The syndrome of the region of the supramarginal gyrus (zone B) consists of anarthria and aphasia with weakness of the arm, hemianesthesia, sometimes bilateral apraxia, and no hemianopsia. Lesions in the region of the angular gyrus and the posterior part of the first two temporal convolutions (zone C) are

68

characterized by alexia, agraphia, hemianopsia, difficulty in comprehension, in calculation, and in naming, but no anarthria, weakness, or sensory loss. The syndrome of the temporal region (zone D) consists of inability to name (loss of vocabulary), difficulty in comprehension of speech, in reading, in writing and in

HEAD'S TYPES OF APHASIA

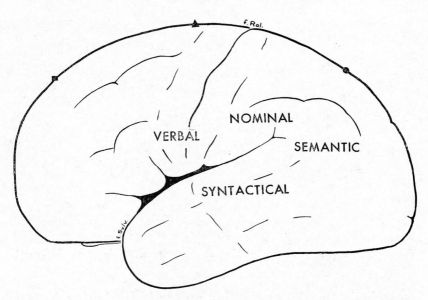

FIG. IV-5. A brain map to show locations of the lesions in the types of aphasia, as described by Henry Head (1926).

calculating, diminished intelligence, hemianopsia, but no anarthria or hemiplegia. And, finally, a lesion in zone E produces anarthria and aphasia of profound degree associated with hemiplegia and a certain degree of hemianesthesia.

Wilson (1926) gave a clear, concise exposition on aphasia which embodied the theory of association areas with only cortical connections. He stated that aphasia is, physiologically, a disorder of transcortical mechanisms (Jackson's highest level) which play on those of the cortical projection class (Jackson's middle level). Actually, it seems that Wilson was accepting most of the old concepts of localization and of thinking with words alone (not heeding Head's emphasis that a word, phrase, sentence, or even a paragraph may not be meaningful except as part of the total idea).

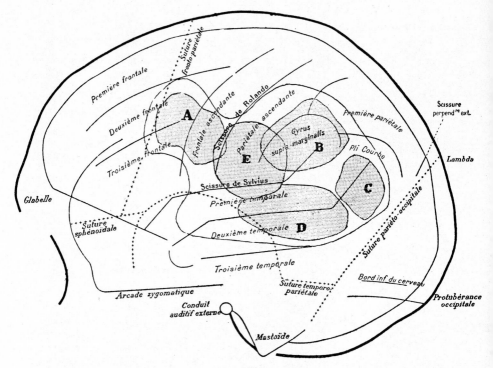

FIG. IV-6. A map to show the location of the zones of Marie and Foix (1917), see text.

Goldstein (1948) began writing on aphasia shortly after the turn of the century and continued for over forty years. He applied the principles of Gestalt psychology to the study of brain lesions. He stressed the "loss of the abstract with retention of the concrete" and the avoidance of what he termed "catastrophic conditions" for the aphasic.

Von Kuenburg (1930) demonstrated in her testing of classification of colors and objects that normal behavior is not controlled always by "categorical principle." *Meyers* (1948) found no statistical difference in the ability to solve a multiple choice problem between patients with receptive aphasia, those with lesions of the non-dominant hemisphere, and those with lesions of the spinal cord and peripheral nerves. It does not seem that the problems of aphasia have been solved by the Gestalt psychologists. Also, Goldstein's (1948) eight cases with autopsy had such diffuse lesions that they are of little value in anatomical localization.

Weisenburg and *McBride* (1935) criticized some of Head's (1926) tests on the basis that they cannot be done by all normal subjects. They presented an excellently controlled study. They stated that aphasia is divided into four groups: predominantly expressive, predominantly receptive, expressive-receptive, and amnesic. Gross or diffuse lesions were present in their cases.

Nielsen (1936-1953) is the current champion of the precise localization school (Fig. IV-7).

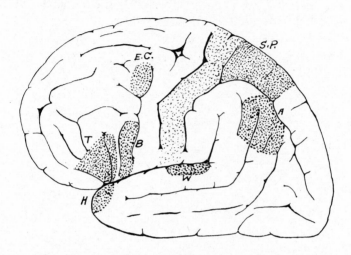

Fig. IV-7. A map of the important areas for speech as outlined by Nielsen (1946). T represents the motor center for music; B, Broca's area; E.C., the writing center; H, Henschen's auditory music center; W, Wernicke's area; A, angular gyrus; and S.P., the superior parietal region.

Schiller (1947) summarized a study of forty-six convalescent cases of penetrating missile wounds. He listed "articulation, inflection, bradyphasia, paraphasia, jargon, telegram, syntax, perseveration, nominal, auditory comprehension, visual comprehension, spelling, construction, calculation, and apraxia;" and he stated that disorders of the former half of the list give place to those of the latter half as the site of the wound becomes more posterior. Nominal aphasia was present in almost all cases, regardless of location of injury. He suggested a classification as frontal, fronto-temporal, etc., types of aphasia.

Sachs (1905) and *Guttman* (1942) emphasized that aphasia does occur in children, the youngest patient being about two years old.

Critchley (1938) reported "aphasia" in a partial deaf-mute and demonstrated the deficiency in the use of sign language.

Each author's theories and observations cannot be given, but we should like to mention the following contributors: Hammond (1871), Cross (1872), Barlow (1877), Ball (1881), Heilly and Chantemese (1883), Bernard (1885), Hartmann (1889), Starr (1889), Freud (1891), Gowers (1893), Shaw (1893), Elder (1897), Bramwell (1898), Bernheim (1900), Bianchi (1910), Smith (1917-18), Kleist (1934), Zucker (1934), Kennedy and Wolf (1936), Klein (1937), Lhermitte (1937), Austregesilo (1940), Cobb (1943), Teitelbaum (1943), Alajouanine (1948), Alford (1948), Ajuria-guerra and Hécaen (1949), Bay (1952), Zeigler (1952), Critchley (1953), and Conrad (1951).

In summary, much has been learned about aphasia since Broca's time. It would seem that most authors agree that lesions in specific localities produce definite clinical types of aphasia. The closer the lesion is to Broca's area (the posterior part of the third frontal convolution) and the adjacent precentral face area, the more the motor components of speech are involved. The nearer the lesion is to the vicinity of the junction of the parietal, temporal and occipital lobes, the more reading and writing are affected; and the more the posterior superior temporal region is involved, the greater the difficulty in the comprehension of spoken words. Head's (1926) warning that there are no fundamental individual faculties of speech, reading, and writing should be heeded; but until a better classification of the dysphasias is forthcoming, the disorders of speech, reading, and writing should be recorded.

Lesions restricted to small areas such as Broca's area are extremely rare. The best examples of so-called "pure" disturbances such as "pure motor aphasia" are clinical descriptions without pathological correlations (e.g. Nielsen, 1936b). In most if not all of the reported cases, discrete lesions have resulted in only transient aphasia.

As far as the recorded literature is concerned, the difference in the clinical syndrome produced by lesions of the precentral motor face area as compared with lesions of Broca's area is extremely difficult to ascertain because of the scarcity of cases with a lesion limited to one or the other area, or lack of microscopic identification of the areas, or insufficient clinical data.

Difficulty in naming, also perseveration, are recorded in practically all cases of aphasia. In the large posterior lesions, which were found in most of the cases in the literature, reading and writing seem to be affected more than the understanding of spoken language. In most of these cases the lesions are not discrete but seem to have involved parts of the parietal, temporal, and occipital lobes.

B. *On agnosia and apraxia*

Agnosia. In 1876, *Hughlings Jackson* described a 59-year-old woman who two months before admission to hospital suddenly lost her way and was unable to get home from the nearby park. When she did reach home she seemed normal. But from then on she would do odd things such as put sugar in her tea two or three times or put her clothes on backwards. Three weeks later she became unconscious and remained so for forty-eight hours. It was noticed then that her left arm and leg were paralyzed. She gradually improved but mistook the identities of people about her. She was unable to read Snellen's chart, but started at the right lower corner and read: "The name colony" and "name" again. At the end of the line she did not know where to go; at last she pointed to "the" and said, "That's 'the' and to me they look all the's, the's, the's." She named familiar objects. A fortnight later no mental imperfection could be demonstrated. Then she suddenly became unresponsive and died the same day. At autopsy multiple gliomatous tumors were found in the right temporo-occipital region. This condition Jackson called partial *imperception*.

In 1883, *Charcot* (1890, vol. 3, pp. 178-193) described a patient with loss of visual memory of objects and persons and of certain letters (which he recognized only after tracing them himself). As previously noted, Bastian had already described word-blindness and word-deafness. Lissauer (1890) considered that perception was divided into conscious perception of sensory impressions—apperception—and linkage of content of perception with other images—association. *Freud* (1891) introduced the term *agnosia* to apply to loss of association (second stage of Lissauer).

Goldstein and Gelb (1918) reported in great detail the visual disturbances in one patient; they considered him to have apperceptive mind-blindness, which was not due to the loss of memory images in the association field, but to loss of figure-ground relationship or visual Gestalten. As several authors have pointed out, they did not demonstrate vision to be normal in the remaining fields.

The term agnosia has been given a number of different meanings by various authors. Visual verbal agnosia has been considered the same as word-blindness. Dejerine (1914) maintained that "pure word-blindness" is caused by a lesion of the angular gyrus. The literature has been reviewed to determine if such a condition can be found, but no case seems to meet these requirements. The nearest approach to "pure word-blindness" occurred in a patient who showed at autopsy an occipital lobe infarction, reported by Henshelwood.* However, the clinical examination was incomplete. Even Nielsen (1946) did not present cases to prove his statement that visual verbal (or literal or numerical) agnosia is produced by a lesion of the angular gyrus.

Bastian first used the term word-deafness, and this has been stated to be equivalent to auditory verbal agnosia. Nielsen (1946) considered that one hears sounds and "stores up memory pictures (develops engrams) of certain words (utilizes the function of auditory eugnosia). Physiologically speaking, there are two levels of integration: primary perception and eugnosia. Destruction of the first results in deafness; of the second, in agnosia—acoustic or auditory agnosia if complete, acoustic verbal agnosia if recognition of words only is lost. . . . A patient may become sound deaf so that he does not hear anything; he then has lost primary perception. He may, however, retain ability to hear sounds but lose the ability to recognize that he had heard them before. Or he may retain memory of having heard general sounds before but not the memory of having heard sounds of words before. The anatomic site of formation of engrams of words is therefore different from that of other sounds." (p. 25)

Nielsen then stated that the first transverse gyri of Heschl on both sides are devoted to hearing; Wernicke's area (posterior half of the first and part of the second temporal convolutions) is the center of auditory recognition. Lesions, he said, which produce auditory verbal agnosia have to interrupt the fiber tracts from both

---

* The summary of this case is taken from Weisenburg and McBride, 1935, page 66; and Henschen, 1920, case 155.

hearing centers to Wernicke's center, or the lesion must destroy the latter on the dominant side.

If the preceding were true, then a lesion involving peripheral auditory pathways could not produce any form of auditory verbal agnosia. Schuknecht and Woellner (1955) have shown that essentially normal, pure-tone thresholds for the speech frequencies (512, 1024, and 2048 c.p.s.) may exist with a speech discrimination score of only sixteen per cent in a patient who had an acoustic neurinoma. In other words a lesion which has incompletely destroyed the auditory nerve may result in the patient being able to appreciate pure tones (which is usually the only thing tested in routine audiometry) but not being able to reproduce speech sounds.

In reviewing the cases of "word-deafness," one is unable to find a single case with an isolated defect. There are cases in which comprehension of speech is the most involved, but none of these cases shows conclusively that hearing is intact. Miller (1950) has found no case of "congenital auditory imperception," as repeated audiometric tests have shown considerable partial deafness in all. "In some of them the failure of understanding speech seems disproportionate to degree of hearing deficit which in other subjects is not accompanied by such a pronounced failure of understanding, but this is a far cry from attributing the defect wholly to a specific agnosia of cortical origin."

In the case of Henschen (1920, No. 3), on which Nielsen laid great stress, there was complete involvement of Wernicke's zone bilaterally without producing complete loss of understanding speech. The lesions which have produced the difficulty in understanding involved both temporal regions, usually the first and second temporal, and Heschl's convolutions—cases summarized by Mills (1891), Barrett (1910), and Henschen (1918).

Lissauer's theory of perception and Nielsen's concept of eugnosia with its anatomical localizations are not satisfactory. Nor is agnosia valid when based upon such notions.

Progress has been retarded by the assumption that "primary" vision is intact in such a patient. If the size of the letters is increased, frequently the patient will be able to read what he could not read in normal-sized letters. This may be true even though the visual acuity and examination by perimetry and campimmetry are normal.

By definition, visual verbal agnosia means inability to recognize a word by sight, vision being within normal limits. When one reads about such a case, it is immediately apparent that the patient did recognize some words, and many words at some time. The variability of the response is obvious, as emphasized by many.

Bay (1951) has shown that, experimentally, visual agnosia can be produced by dimming the light, limiting the visual field, etc. There is no evidence that perception is divided into "apperception and association." More refined tests such as those used by Teuber and Bender (1948), and Bay (1950, 1953) for visual perception, and those of Schubert and Panse (1953), and Schuknecht and Woellner (1955) for auditory perception, must be used. We agree with Reinhold (1954) that final perception occurring at a single moment in time is a multidimensional experience.

Varieties of defective perception may be called various types of agnosia; however, it would be better to return to Hughlings Jackson's term of *imperception* which does not have the theoretical connotations that Freud's *agnosia* does. Only after further research, carried out in man with the same meticulousness as it is in animals, will we have a more acceptable theory of perception.

Apraxia. Again *Jackson* (1931) was first to describe the inability of a patient to put out his tongue upon request, even though he knew what was desired and later would stick it out automatically to lick his lips. This has come to be known as apraxia of the tongue. Although Steinthal and Gogol used the term apraxia, Leipmann in 1900 made a comprehensive analysis of apraxia and clearly distinguished this condition from agnosia (Ajuriaguerra and Hécaen, 1949). Various types of apraxia (kinesthetic, ideo-kinesthetic, ideational, constructional, etc.) have been described; but let us consider only the concepts held by Wilson (1926), Nielsen (1946), and others that motor aphasia is an apraxia of speech, and that of Nielsen (1948), contending that motor aphasia (apraxia of speech) and agraphia (apraxia of writing) are produced by lesions of the posterior parts of the third and second frontal convolutions, respectively.

Of the forty-three cases Nielsen (1946) presented to support the contention that the destruction of Broca's area produces motor aphasia, there is not a single case which is convincing; either the case was incompletely reported clinically or pathologically, or the clinical and pathological findings were incongruous (e.g. hemi-plegia with only a lesion of the third frontal convolution), or there was no aphasia. The case of Scheinker and Kuhr (1948) is unsatis-factory because of the acuteness of the lesion. There is one case reported by Banti (Bastian, 1898; and Henschen, 1922, case 727) of a 36-year-old man who had a right hemiparesis and loss of speech. The hemiparesis disappeared quickly, but he was com-pletely mute, though able to write correctly and rapidly and to understand oral and written directions. A little over four years later it was stated that he had almost completely recovered speech by re-education, though when this happened was not indicated. At autopsy there was a lesion limited to the posterior part of the left third frontal convolution. Of all the cases reported in the literature, here is one that seems to fit the criteria! And there was recovery.

There is also one case to support the thesis of a "writing center" in the second frontal convolution. Gordinier (1899) reported a 37-year-old woman who for three months had had headaches, vomiting, and failing vision. She had papilledema and weakness of the right hand (though fine movements were present) and a right sixth cranial nerve paresis. She could speak, read, name, and understand speech. She was unable to write with either hand— however, from the samples given, some letters are easily recogniz-able. Over the next six weeks she became slow in speech, though not aphasic, and she tended to fall to the right. Trepanation was carried out and no tumor was seen. She died two days later. There was a glioma two centimeters in length at the foot of the second frontal convolution, extending to the ventricle and invading the white matter of the first frontal gyrus. The cerebral hernia which followed the operation involved the precentral gyrus. Again, the lesion was not a static one but was progressive over a period of only three months and eventually caused death.

Jackson believed that within Broca's region were represented movements of tongue, palate, lips, larynx, and pharynx. We now know that stimulation of the precentral gyrus yields such move-ments. As will be shown later, electrical arrest in Broca's area yields the same kinds of alteration in speech as does electrical arrest in the parietal and temporal regions. If the patient is not attempting to speak, no words are evoked from stimulation of Broca's area; nor, as a rule, are any movements of swallowing, etc. noted.

If engrams of motor speech were stored in Broca's area, as *Nielsen* (1946) has suggested, one might expect that words might be produced by stimulation. Nielsen's concept—that with a lesion of the Betz cells, paralysis would result; that with a lesion of the cells just anterior to the Betz cells "which are utilized for movements of the head, especially for the mouth, the patient would forget how to make accurate movements with the mouth;" and that if the cells "still farther forward which are necessary for speech were affected, motor aphasia would result,"* has never been substantiated. Just as the theories behind agnosia must be modified, so must those of apraxia.

C. *On localization*

No discrete localization of lesions producing various types of agnosia and apraxia has been found. It seems, as *Jackson* (1931) stated, that any acute lesion to any gross part of the left hemisphere will produce some disturbance in speech. It should be mentioned that this includes disease of the anterior (Critchley, 1930) and posterior (Brown-Séquard, 1877) cerebral arteries as well as of the middle cerebral.

Magnan (1879), Elsberg (1931), Cushing and Eisenhardt (1938), Poppen (1939), Erickson and Woolsey (1951), and Chusid et al. (1954) have reported dysphasia accompanying tumors involving the medial and superior aspects of the posterior part of the left first frontal convolution. Most of these tumors were comparatively small meningeal ones. Liepman and Maas (1907), Critchley (1930), Hyland (1933), Ethelburg (1951), and Petit-Dutaillis et al. (1954) have reported disturbances in speech with disorders of circulation of the anterior cerebral arteries. When the disease involved the right anterior cerebral artery, the disorder was a dysarthric one; but dysphasic defects have been noted when the lesion was on the left. The articulatory disturbances have been attributed by Ethelburg to a general "disorder of rapid and complex movements."

From the studies of patients with frontal lobectomies and lobotomies, it is clear that all of the frontal lobe anterior to Broca's

---

* Nielsen (1946, page 28).

area may be removed without permanent aphasia. Burckhardt (1891) claimed that he removed part of Broca's area without aphasia. Mettler (1949) stated that all of Broca's area may be removed bilaterally without aphasia. As the motor cortex was not outlined by stimulation, and as no case has been reported with autopsy performed, this statement is doubtful. Nor did Jefferson (1950) state how he determined Broca's area when he mentioned that "excisions of Broca's area, with care to avoid deep undercuts in the white matter, have led at most to nothing more than transient aphasia."

As *Nielsen* (1948) pointed out, there are a number of cases in the literature with destruction of the left Broca's area without aphasia. *Nielsen* (1948, page 571) stated: "There is no case on record of bilateral destruction of Broca's convolution* with retained ability to speak." From the standpoint of gross anatomy, there is such a case. This case (#41 of Moutier, 1908) is that of a 75-year-old woman who had right hemiplegia and aphasia at the age of 73. Speech returned, and at the age of 75 she had another stroke with left hemiplegia. Prior to death she was definitely able to speak. There was bilateral destruction of the posterior part of the third frontal convolution, exclusive of other lesions. However, the brain was not examined microscopically. There is another case (#260 of Moutier, 1908) in which the entire left Broca's area was destroyed, but the small postero-superior part of the right third frontal convolution was intact.

Burckhardt (1891) removed the posterior parts of the first and second temporal convolutions without permanent aphasia. Wernicke's area may be involved bilaterally without complete loss of ability to understand spoken language (Henschen, 1918).

Bilateral destruction of the lenticular nucleus without difficulty in speech was reported (Nielsen, 1946). It is unknown whether isolated lesions of the thalamus are accompanied by aphasia. Smyth and Stern (1938) reported no speech disturbance with tumors of the ventral nuclear group of the thalamus; but they found marked speech and mental disturbances with tumors of the medial and anterior thalamic nuclei. Kubik and Adams (1946)

---

* Nielsen (1948) defined Broca's convolution as limited posteriorly by the precentral gyrus, anteriorly by the pars triangularis, and superiorly by the second frontal gyrus—in other words, the one gyrus anterior to the precentral face area.

found dysarthria and mental confusion with occlusion of the basilar artery, without involvement of the posterior cerebral. It is not clear whether the cases of Smyth and Stern and those of Kubik and Adams should be classed as aphasic. Brown-Séquard (1877) stated that aphasia (not just a motor disturbance) was noted with pontine lesions, but he did not present the material upon which this opinion was based; nor have similar cases been presented since.

The speech areas of practically all authors include the posterior inferior part of the frontal lobe, the posterior half of the first and second temporal gyri, the angular gyrus, and the temporo-

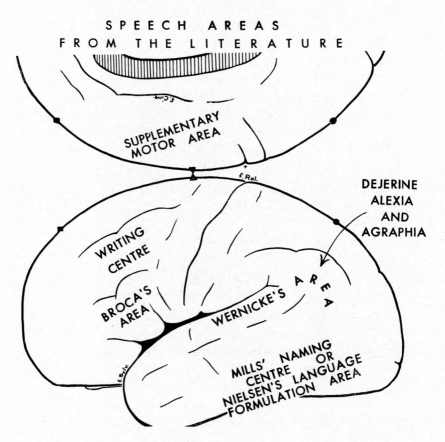

SPEECH AREAS
FROM THE LITERATURE

Fig. IV-8. Summary of some of the important areas for speech as described in the literature. The writing center was first described by Wernicke and later by Exner. The supplementary motor area was first described by Penfield, and Roberts (1952) showed what its relation to speech might be.

DISORDERS OF SPEECH
FROM THE LITERATURE

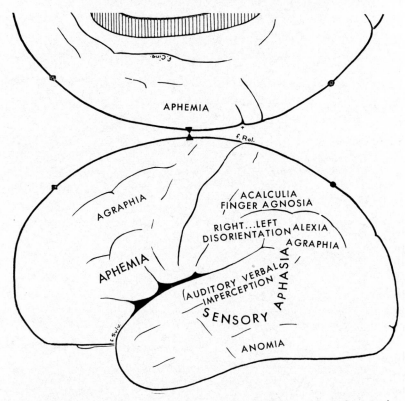

Fig. IV-9. Summary of the location of the lesion which could produce various disorders of speech as noted in the literature. Petit-Dutaillis et al. stated that aphemia occurs with lesions of the supplementary motor area, which was described by Penfield.

parieto-occipital junction (Figs. IV-8 and IV-9). None of the theories of the various types of aphasia have had general acceptance. Despite a century of study, the mechanisms of speech and aphasia remain as challenging problems.

CHAPTER V

METHODS OF INVESTIGATION

L. R.

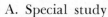

A. Special study
B. The sodium amytal aphasia test
C. Disturbances in speech with seizures

DISTURBANCES in speech with seizures, the results of electrical identification of cortical speech areas, the results of cortical excision with the evolution of transient aphasia during the post-operative period, similar studies when the non-dominant hemisphere was involved, studies of handedness and of cerebral dominance (including the sodium amytal aphasia test)—all these things constitute the material of this study. Of greatest interest are those patients who had excisions carried out in what the surgeon considered the close vicinity of speech areas of the dominant hemisphere.

The surgical excision of cerebral cortex in the treatment of focal cerebral seizures demands of the neurosurgeon that he should study localization of function in each case with great care. He must learn to respect areas of brain, the function of which is essential, or to sacrifice, knowingly, areas which are dispensable. When it becomes necessary to consider ablation of cortex in the vicinity of cortical speech areas, the problem of the exact limits of those areas used for speech becomes a critical one.

The studies and these cases are reconsidered now to see what light may be thrown concerning those areas necessary for speech. The records of all patients operated on for seizures from 1928 through February 6, 1951 have been reviewed for evidence of disturbance in speech during stimulation and for evidence of aphasia before and after operation. Five hundred and sixty-nine patients had 663 operations, about fifty per cent involving each hemisphere. Attempts to arrest or interfere with speech by electrical interference were made in 190 cases—121 involving the left hemisphere and 69, the right.

A. *Special study*

A special study of seventy-two patients* was carried out before and, periodically, after operation for evidence of dysphasia. The seventy-two patients are divided into four groups, as follows: operations on the left hemisphere—with language disturbances, 26; without language disturbance, 19; and operations on the right hemisphere—with language disturbance, 1; without language disturbance, 26.

The following special tests have been applied to this series of seventy-two patients before and, periodically, after operation.

Spontaneous speech includes the understanding of speech as well as the control of speaking. No patient was found to be completely speechless. None gave evidence of understanding nothing.

The degree of deficit was judged subjectively by the examiner employing the words 1) questionable, 2) slight, 3) moderate, 4) marked, and 5) very marked. These five grades of disturbance of spontaneous speech were recorded, in proportion to the increasing amount of deficit, as 1, 2, 3, 4, and 5. The degree of difficulty in perseveration, naming, etc. was recorded numerically also.

Perseveration is used to mean the uncontrolled repetition of words or nonsense sounds during spontaneous speech. It may appear also during naming tests. Perseveration has been judged subjectively.

Naming. The following were named routinely: 12 objects (key, pencil, match, scissors, comb, spoon, safety pin, thumb tack, paper clip, quarter, dime, and nickel); 8 miniature objects (chair, stove, pipe, boot, watch, cat, telephone, and spoon); and 21 small pictures (bird, comb, knife, horse, bed, tree, drum, apple, house, butterfly, table, top, hat, foot, clock, fish, glove, scissors, cow, hammer, and flag).

Some patients failed to name one or more of the preceding before operation; the thumb tack, paper clip, coins (by foreigners), boot, butterfly, or top were the objects missed. Frequently the patient could describe rather accurately the use of the object but could not put the concrete name to it; or he might call the boot a shoe, or the butterfly a moth. Failure to name one or two of these

* Three of these patients were examined by Mr. Robert Sparks, then speech pathologist at the Royal Victoria Hospital and the Montreal Neurological Institute.

objects is classed as a questionable defect (1); failure to name one-fourth of them is slight difficulty (2); one-half, moderate difficulty (3); three-fourths, marked difficulty (4); and more than three-fourths is classed as very marked difficulty in naming (5). Immediately, and for the first few days after operation, the patient was asked to name only about ten objects (usually the first ten small pictures); as soon as feasible, all objects were used again.

Repetition includes the repeating of "Methodist Episcopal," "British Constitution," "The Third Riding Artillery Brigade," and "Around the rugged rock the ragged rascal ran." Also the patient is asked to repeat "key, pencil, match, scissors, comb, and spoon" as a unit. If he cannot do the preceding, he is classed as having marked difficulty in repetition and is requested to repeat individual words.

Oral commands consist of asking the patient to put his right second finger on his left ear, or his left third finger on his right eyebrow, etc. If the patient can do none of these commands he is said to have very marked difficulty in obeying commands, and is given simpler ones. If he obeys some of these commands, he is given two, then three of the preceding simultaneously. If the patient fails on the three simultaneous commands and executes the others, he is classified as having slight difficulty. If he obeys one-half of the two simultaneous commands, he has moderate difficulty; and if he obeys none of them but obeys the single commands, he has marked difficulty.

Written commands consist of the same type as the oral commands described, e.g. "Put your left third finger on your right eyebrow." Only two commands similar to the preceding are given together as a unit, and if not obeyed, the patient has slight difficulty obeying written commands. If he obeys none of the single commands, he has marked difficulty and is given such commands as "Show me your teeth," or "Show me your right second finger." If these are not obeyed, he has very marked difficulty obeying written commands.

Spelling is judged by both oral and written ability; as the writing (see under "spontaneous writing") varies considerably, difficulty in spelling is classified as slight, moderate, marked, and very marked, on a subjective basis.

Reading aloud involves the reading of letters, numbers, words, and simple sentences. As practically all patients before operation read these correctly, this scoring is based on reading the following three sentences* aloud: 1) The test is applicable to individuals above the 8 or 9 year level. 2) In explaining each test to the patient use only the phrases given above the form. 3) Repeat each test three times and in the same sequence.

In the immediate period after operation only the simple sentences are given, and the difficulty is charted on the basis of the percentage of the whole missed. At times there is a difference in the ability to read numbers as compared with letters and words, and this is noted. As soon as feasible the more difficult reading is given.

Silent reading consists of reading and repeating the following three sentences: 1) Do not help the patient out. 2) Be sure to record verbatim all hesitations and incorrect responses. 3) A pause is to be judged as such depending on the mental activity of the patient. Scoring is made on the following basis: Each sentence counts thirty-three and one-third per cent, with the actual words counting one-half and the meaning, one-half. If the meaning is not clear to the examiner, questions are asked and both questions and answers recorded. No time limit is set. If the patient cannot repeat anything, three simpler sentences are used: 1) Snow is cold. 2) Bread is good to eat. 3) The man and his dog went for a walk in the woods.

Spontaneous writing. The patient is given writing materials and asked to write a page on a subject of his own choosing. There is considerable variation and the scoring is on a subjective basis.

Writing to dictation includes writing the words and sentences, which are the same as those used in repetition.

Copying. The patient is asked to copy words that are shown him in written form.

Oral calculation includes the following problems: 8 plus 4, 29 plus 36, 100 minus 7, 18 from 34, 8 times 4, 9 times 7, 13 times 13, 8 divided by 4, 36 divided by 6, 96 divided by 6, and 256

---

* These three sentences and those below under "silent reading" were instructions for the examiner in the "Modified Chesher Test" used at the Montreal Neurological Institute; nonetheless, they were given to these patients.

divided by 16. If the simpler problem in each category is not answered correctly, others even simpler are given. This test is not repeated until thought feasible after operation.

Written calculation includes the following problems: 863 + 136, 864 + 958, 986 − 121, 988 − 889, 4567 − 5456, 94 × 37, 9.08 × 95, 48048 ÷ 24, and 64064 ÷ 32. Simpler problems are given if required.

The preceding tests have been given by the writer. In other examinations and in general neurological tests we have been assisted by various members of the staff of the Montreal Neurological Institute.

B. *The sodium amytal aphasia test*

Wada (1949) introduced a valuable procedure for determining which hemisphere subserves speech. Sodium amytal is injected into the carotid artery while the patient is counting and making rapidly alternating movements of the fingers of both hands. If the drug has been injected into either the common or internal carotid artery, there is a contralateral hemiplegia. The patient usually stops counting.

If the non-dominant hemisphere is involved, the subject usually begins to count again after a brief pause. During the period of silence, the patient is more or less confused, generally with brief loss of contact with environment. As a rule, counting is recommenced in less than thirty seconds. He is able to speak, to name, and to read correctly. There may be somatic and visual sensory loss contralaterally. The hemiplegia disappears gradually in about five minutes. Afterwards the patient denies the hemiplegia.

If the dominant hemisphere is involved, the patient remains silent for one minute or so. He then may be confused in his counting, or he may count correctly but show difficulty in naming and in reading with the use of nonsense, perseveration, and miscalling. Frequently the hemiplegia clears before his speech returns to normal. Usually the patient admits the hemiplegia.

We have used this test at the Montreal Neurological Institute in those cases, particularly the left-handed, in which surgical therapy of seizures was contemplated where the lesion was in the region of a speech area if the hemisphere was dominant for speech.

A preliminary report has been made by Rasmussen and Wada (1959).

It should be pointed out that the electroencephalogram usually shows only ipsilateral abnormalities, but occasionally there are bilateral disturbances, particularly in the contralateral frontal region. The latter probably means that the drug has crossed into the opposite hemisphere through the circle of Willis.

This test has been interpreted to show that speech was represented unilaterally in all but three cases. These three cases showed a pronounced disturbance in speech with one injection, and only a very questionable difficulty with the other. In addition, following operation involving the hemisphere where equivocal disturbance in speech had occurred with the sodium amytal test in two cases, no difficulty in speech was detected. In the third case, transient dysphasia occurred after operation involving the hemisphere where definite disturbance in speech had occurred with this test. Probably speech was not represented bilaterally in these cases either. However, bilateral representation of speech remains a possibility.

C. *Disturbances in speech with seizures*

Both positive and negative effects on speech may occur with seizures. The positive effect—vocalization—occurs with epileptic discharge in the Rolandic or supplementary motor area of either hemisphere or in subcortical regions. The negative effects are several. The patient may be unable to understand what is said to him. This inability to comprehend can be interference with primary auditory mechanisms or with speech mechanisms. With the latter the patient states that he knows that someone is speaking, since he can hear the words but is unable to comprehend. The discharge is in the dominant hemisphere. Epileptic discharge producing interference with primary auditory mechanisms can be in either hemisphere or in subcortical regions. At times it is not possible to ascertain whether it is speech or primary audition which is affected.

If the patient is reading when he has a seizure, there may be a disturbance in reading. Again, this may be a primary visual disturbance or one in speech. In the latter case he may read incorrectly with dysphasic mistakes, and the discharge would be in the dominant hemisphere, whereas in the former it can be in either hemisphere or in subcortical regions. Because of the short duration of the epileptic discharge, it may be impossible to distinguish the two, even if the patient is examined during an attack, for the evidence may be all subjective without any objective data.

The patient may be unable to speak in a seizure. If one can establish that contact with environment has not been lost, then the disturbance in speech may be either a pure motor disturbance or a dysphasic one. Motor disturbance may occur with seizure discharges in either Rolandic or supplementary motor area of either hemisphere. Dysphasic disturbances occur with seizures involving a speech area of the dominant hemisphere. If there is silence, then one does not know if the discharge is in motor or speech areas. If there is dysarthric speech, one again does not know if discharge is in motor or speech areas. When there is misnaming or perseveration, the discharge is in a speech area.

On rare occasion a seizure may occur while the patient is writing, and there may be dysgraphic disturbances if the discharge is in a speech area.

The disturbances in language may occur as an aura, during the seizure, or postictally. Disturbances in comprehension, reading, motor speech, or writing may occur with seizures originating in the temporo-parietal or Broca's or supplementary motor area of the dominant hemisphere. The focus of the seizure discharge may be adjacent to a speech area in so-called silent areas of cortex; the electroencephalogram can be helpful in establishing that the electrographic discharge began not in a speech area but adjacent to it.

CHAPTER VI

HANDEDNESS AND CEREBRAL DOMINANCE

L. R.

A. Literature
B. Analysis of our cases
C. Discussion
    1. On aphasia
    2. On handedness
    3. On shift of dominance
D. Summary

A. *Literature*

Marc Dax found lesions of the left hemisphere in forty cases in which there had been a disturbance in speech during life. This fact was unknown in Paris in 1861 when Broca published his first case. Broca (1863) pointed out that nineteen of twenty cases with aphemia had lesions of the left hemisphere; however, he was cautious about making any generalization.

Dax's lecture was again presented in 1863, this time in Paris by his son. In the discussions on the "Faculté du Langage Articulé" at the Royal Academy of Medicine in 1865, *Bouillaud* correlated the fact that aphasia occurs with lesions of the left cerebral hemisphere with the fact that most people are right-handed.

Some weeks later *Broca* summarized a case reported by Moreau the year before: a 47-year-old woman had had epilepsy and right hemiparesis since infancy. She was left-handed. At no time had there been any speech disturbance. At autopsy there was a large lesion in the distribution of the left middle cerebral artery. Broca assumed, and we believe correctly, that speech had been subserved by the right hemisphere in this patient. He then went on to generalize unjustifiably that the right hemisphere is dominant for speech in all of the left-handed. Thus was created the dogma that the *right cerebral hemisphere* is dominant for speech in the *left-handed* in the same way that the *left cerebral hemisphere* is supposed to be for the *right-handed.*

89

Handedness was not mentioned in the literature prior to 1865. *Hughlings Jackson* (1864) reported three cases with left hemiplegia and thirty-one with right hemiplegia; all thirty-four had loss of speech. Four years later he mentioned that one of these patients with left hemiplegia was not left-handed but right-handed, but he did not give the handedness of the other two. In the same article Jackson reported the first case of a left-handed man with a lesion of the right hemisphere and aphasia—he seems to have accepted Broca's and Bouillaud's theory, and it is doubtful that Jackson realized that his was the first positive case reported, as the theory seemed a good one.

The literature has been reviewed from the standpoint of presence or absence of aphasia in the left-handed and ambidextrous with unilateral cerebral disease. Also a search has been made to determine the handedness of all cases reported to have aphasia with involvement of only the right hemisphere.

A number of investigators have pointed out that the greater the number of tests used, the fewer become the number of purely left- or right-handed. Those individuals who were stated to do most things, including writing, with their right hand are classed as right-handed. Those individuals who generally use their left hand but who use their right hand for writing, and perhaps other acts, are classed as predominantly left-handed (practically all of the ambidextrous cases are included here). Most of the cases in the left-handed group have been recorded by authors as left-handed, with no details provided concerning the right hand.

Aphasia has been reported with involvement of the right hemisphere in 136 patients. Handedness was as follows: right, 53;[1] left, 42;[2] predominantly left, 23;[3] and unknown or not recorded, 18.[4]

[1] Cases of Bruce (1868); Jackson (1868, 1880), 2 cases; Heine (1903); Mollard (1903, from Oppenheim 1913); Senator (1904); Mills and Weisenburg (1905); Meyer, S. (1908); Meyer, W. (1909); Souques (1910); Lewandowsky (1911); Mendel (1912, from Ludwig 1938); Oppenheim (1913), 2 cases; Raggi (1915, from Ardin-Delteil et al. 1923); Kennedy (1916); Stauffenberg (1918); Henschen (1920 #28 and #29), 2 cases; Claude and Schaeffer (1921, from Ardin-Delteil et al. 1923); Ardin-Delteil et al. (1923); Wilson (1926); Knjaizinskij (1927, from Ludwig 1938); Spalke (1927, from Ludwig 1938); Lovell et al. (1932); Dimitri (1933); Stone (1934); Weisenburg and McBride (1935), 2 cases; Chesher (1936); Ludwig (1938), 7 cases; Marinescu et al. (1938); Humphrey and Zangwill (1952a); Subirana (1952), 2 cases; Ettlinger et al. (1955), including Whitty (unpublished), 2 cases; and Semmes (1956), 10 cases.

[2] Cases of Jackson (1868); Ogle (1871), 3 cases; Habershon (1880); Banti (1886, from Henschen 1920 #579); Hecht (1887, from Critchley 1954); White (1887);

Following disease of the left hemisphere, aphasia has been noted in 32 left-handed[5] and in 34 predominantly left-handed.[6] In the left-handed it has been noted that aphasia did not occur with lesions in areas which are usually accompanied by speech disturbances: 17 times when disease involved the left side,[7] and 13 times when it was the right hemisphere.[8] Similarly, aphasia did not occur except twice when the left hemisphere was involved,[9] and six times when it was the right half[10] in the predominantly left-handed.

Köster (1889); Bell (1895); Runeburg (1896); Rothman (1907); Mingazini (1910, from Henschen 1922 #1101); Sträussler (1911, from Henschen 1920 #482); Seiler, (1913, from Henschen 1920 #313); Dejerine (1914), 3 cases; Taterka (1924); Head (1926); Herman and Pötzl (1926, from Critchley 1954—Gerstmann's syndrome); Weisenburg and McBride (1935); Chesher (1936), 2 cases; Brain (1941); Kennedy (1947); Conrad (1949), 7 cases; Humphrey and Zangwill (1952b); Goodglass and Quadfasel (1954), 3 cases; Semmes (1956), 2 cases; and Subirana (1956), 3 cases.

3 Cases of Jackson (1868, 1880), 2 cases; Wadham (1869); Kussmaul (1877); Cuffer (1880); Bernheim (1885); Féré (1885, from Moutier 1908 #321); Tison (1889); Dejerine (1891, from Moutier 1908 #323); Touche (1899); Dejerine and André-Thomas (1912); Souques (1928); Weisenburg and McBride (1935); Chesher (1936), 3 cases; Nielsen (1937); Humphrey and Zangwill (1952a), 3 cases; Goodglass and Quadfasel (1954), 2 cases; Ettlinger et al. (1956).

4 Cases of Jackson (1864, 1868), 2 cases; Trousseau (1865, including Charcot 3, Vulpian 1, Kirks 1, and Peter 1), 7 cases; Bateman (1869); Finkelnberg (1870); Schreiber (1874); Ledouble and Viollet (1879, from Moutier 1908 #327), Drozda (1880, from Henschen 1922 #880); Mesnet (1882); Moltschanow (1897, from Moutier 1908 #331); and Beduschi (Henschen 1922 #750 and #755), 2 cases.

5 Cases of Miyake (1909); Long (1913); Weisenburg and McBride (1935); Nielsen (1937); Conrad (1949), 10 cases; Wepman (1952), 2 cases; Humphrey and Zangwill (1952a); Critchley (1954, including two cases of Gerstmann's syndrome), 8 cases; Goodglass and Quadfasel (1954, including case of Ballantine and White), 2 cases; Chusid et al. (1954); Ettlinger et al. (1956); and Subirana (1956), 3 cases.

6 Cases of Bourneville (1874, from Moutier 1908 #256); Hervey (1874); Paget (1887); Wood (1889); Dickinson (1898, from Bastian 1898); Bramwell (1899); Rothman (1909); Liepman (1912); Kennedy (1916); Ardin-Delteil et al. (1923); Weisenburg and McBride (1935), 2 cases; Chesher (1936), 5 cases; Tilney (1936); Humphrey and Zangwill (1952a), 4 cases; Subirana (1952); Critchley (1954); Goodglass and Quadfasel (1954), 4 cases; Zangwill (1954); and Ettlinger et al. (1956), 5 cases.

7 Cases of Moreau (1864, from Broca 1888); Taylor (1880); Westphal (1884); Chesher (1936); Bucy and Chase (1937); Gardner (1941); Nielsen (1946); Conrad (1949), 5 cases; Critchley (1954), 3 cases; Ettlinger et al. (1956); and Subirana (1956).

8 Cases of Rothman (1907); Hildebrandt (1908, from Critchley 1954); Kennedy (1916), 2 cases; Gardner (1941); Conrad (1949), 5 cases; Critchley (1954); Goodglass and Quadfasel (1954); and Subirana (1956).

9 Cases of Goodglass and Quadfasel (1954); and Ettlinger et al. (1956).

10 Cases of Kennedy (1916); German and Fox (1934); Humphrey and Zangwill (1952a); Critchley (1954); Goodglass and Quadfasel (1954); Ettlinger et al. (1956).

B. *Analysis of our cases*

The records of 569 patients who were operated upon for treatment of focal cerebral seizures have been reviewed for handedness and evidence of aphasia before and after operation.

The handedness of the patient is considered as that hand used more just prior to operation. In most instances the record states that one or the other hand was used; sometimes it is noted that both hands could be used but one was preferred. If the preferred hand was left, then the patient is classed as predominantly left-handed. As far as could be determined, one hand was preferred, even though only slightly, in all "ambidextrous" patients. In forty-seven cases the handedness was not recorded and these cases are excluded. However, it should be noted that in none of these forty-seven did aphasia occur after operation on the right hemisphere.

Detailed questioning as to handedness was done in those patients examined by the writer. The greater the number of questions asked and tests used, the fewer became the number of entirely right- or left-handed, until they were quite exceptional. However, if these patients considered themselves right-handed, for example, they are so listed in the tables to conform with the classification of the other eighty per cent.

Aphasia is defined as that state in which one has difficulty in speech, comprehension of speech, naming, reading, and writing, or any one or more of them; and it is associated with misuse and/or perseveration of words, but is not due to disturbance in the mechanism of articulation (as in pseudo-bulbar palsy) or involvement of peripheral nerves, nor due to general mental insufficiency. A patient is here classed as having aphasia only if it occurred as a result of operation. In other words, if a patient had some sort of speech disturbance before operation and no change following operation, it is considered that the operation itself had no effect upon speech.

Disturbances in articulation only have been noted after operation on either hemisphere; however, none of these cases are classed as having aphasia in subsequent tables.

Those who used the left hand more (left- and predominantly

left-handed) had aphasia much less frequently after operation on the left hemisphere than the right-handed (see Table VI A). How-

TABLE VI A

DIFFERENCE IN PERCENTAGE OF PATIENTS WITH APHASIA
AFTER OPERATION ON LEFT AND RIGHT HEMISPHERE

Hand	Left Hemisphere			Right Hemisphere			Significance[1] of Difference
	Total No.	No. with Aphasia	%	Total No.	No. with Aphasia	%	
R	175	121		252	1		
			69.8			0.4	<.001
R-L[2]	4	4		2	0		
L	48	10		12	2		
			28.3			9.1	.053
L-R[3]	19	9		10	0		
Total	246	144	58.5	276	3	1.1	<.001

[1] Fisher's (1950) exact method of probability
[2] Predominantly right-handed
[3] Predominantly left-handed

ever, many of these patients had right hemiparesis dating from birth or early in life. To exclude the effect that brain injury might have in determining handedness, all cases with brain damage before the age of two years (arbitrarily chosen age) are omitted from Table VI B.

TABLE VI B

DIFFERENCE IN PERCENTAGE OF PATIENTS WITHOUT INJURY BEFORE
TWO YEARS OF AGE AND WITH APHASIA AFTER OPERATION
ON THE LEFT AND RIGHT HEMISPHERE

Hand	Left Hemisphere			Right Hemisphere			Significance of Difference
	Total No.	No. with Aphasia	%	Total No.	No. with Aphasia	%	
R[1]	157	115	73.2	196	1	0.5	<.001
L[2]	18	13	72.2	15	1	6.7	<.001
Total	175	128	73.1	211	2	0.9	<.001

[1] Including predominantly right
[2] Including predominantly left

If the cases with injury in early life are excluded, there is no difference in the incidence of aphasia after operation on the left hemisphere between the left- and right-handed. The left-handed had aphasia about thirteen times as often as the right-handed following operation on the right hemisphere; however, the difference is not statistically significant.

Again with exclusion of those with injury before the age of two years, the left-handed had aphasia about ten times as often after operation on the left hemisphere as after operation on the right half. Statistically, this difference is very significant.

It has been noted that a person may be left- or right-handed despite injury to the hemisphere opposite the preferred hand; and the preferred hand may be weak or clumsy. In many of these cases there is evidence of bilateral cerebral involvement. Despite the fact that the patient is left-handed with weakness of the right hand from early in life, dysphasia may follow operation on the left hemisphere. The right hemisphere is not necessarily dominant for speech, even though the right hemiparesis occurred early in life as a result of damage to the left hemisphere. One must consider this when hemicortisectomy seems indicated; and we believe that the sodium amytal aphasia test (see Chapter V, page 86) should be performed before operation.

Why did so many of our patients with operation on the left hemisphere show transient aphasia? Several days after surgery, aphasia, hemiparesis, neighborhood seizures, etc. may occur. The deficits may occur after the time one would have expected the maximal brain swelling to have passed; therefore, we have used the adjective "neuroparalytic" to describe this edema. The reasons for the large percentage of patients with *neuroparalytic edema* are believed to be related to the length of time the cortex is exposed to air and perhaps to the number of electric stimulations. Only one in ten of the twenty-five per cent who did not have aphasia following surgery involving the left hemisphere demonstrated other evidence of neuroparalytic edema.

C. *Discussion*

1. *On Aphasia*

With the addition of our cases to those in the literature, 78 of 99* left-handed (including predominantly left-handed) had

* These figures exclude our cases of injury before the age of two years, as well

aphasia after injury to the left hemisphere and 66 of 99 had aphasia with involvement of the right half.

In the literature the so-called negative cases have been reported infrequently; there is, therefore, a definite selection of cases. In addition, reports such as that of Ludwig (1938)* have been omitted because his criteria are not clear. He found that aphasia occurred in 100 of 880 right-handers who had war wounds of the right hemisphere.

From our data, transient dysphasia followed operation on the left hemisphere no more frequently in the right-handed (73%) than in the left-handed (72%), provided those with cerebral injury early in life be excluded. In practically all of our cases where there was no transient aphasia, there was no other evidence of neuroparalytic edema. Therefore, in twenty-five per cent of both the right- and left-handed who had operation involving the left hemisphere, no statement can be made as to whether the left hemisphere was or was not dominant for speech. Many of this twenty-five per cent had removal of the frontal or occipital pole or exploration without excision. The other two to three per cent had some evidence of neuroparalytic edema but no dysphasia. This neuroparalytic edema has manifested itself, for example, by transient weakness of the right extremities following removal of the postcentral gyrus. The speech areas might not have been involved in this edema. Therefore, even in these cases one cannot state that the left hemisphere was not dominant for speech, because what was considered by the surgeon as a speech area was not excised in any of these patients.

Also, objection is taken to some of the so-called negative cases in the literature. Case 8 of Ettlinger et al. (1956) is stated to have speech representation on the right because he showed no dysphasia with a glioma of the left half. We have seen similar patients who have later developed dysphasia. Seemingly similar infiltrating tumors in similar locations may show surprisingly different clini-

---

as the cases of Rothman (1909), Moreau (Broca, 1888), Bucy and Chase (1937), and Gardner (1941).

* Cases reported by the following authors have been excluded from this analysis because in the writer's opinion they are not clear: Pye-Smith (1871), Russell (1874), Raymond and Dreyfous (1882), Bouchard (from Bitot, 1884), Pick (1892), Nonne (1899), Spiller (1906), Zilgien (from Moutier, 1908, case #339), Ludwig (1938), Krynauw (1950), Nielsen (1953), and Heuyer and Feld (1954).

cal pictures. We believe that it is not proved that this case of Ettlinger et al. had speech on the right.

In our cases, transient dysphasia following operation on the right hemisphere was not significantly more frequent in the left-handed than in the right-handed. With the addition of our cases to those in the literature, 54 right-handed and 66 left-handed had dysphasia with disease of the right hemisphere. If one considers the ratio of right-to left-handed to be ten to one, then the preceding difference is obviously significant. In part, at least, this is an artifact in the cases selected to be reported, and in the writer's selection, for example, to omit the 100 right-handers of Ludwig (1938). Quadfasel pointed out in discussing a paper by Roberts (1955) that there are about twice as many left-handed as right-handed patients who had dysphasia with disease of the right hemisphere recorded by authors specifically interested in cerebral and hand dominance; again, reports such as Ludwig (1938) are excluded. Nevertheless, if a patient is seen with left hemiplegia and aphasia, "my bookie quotes odds of 12 to 1 that he is left-handed or 1 to 14 that he is right-handed!"

The occurrence of left-handedness in the family of the right-handed who have had dysphasia with involvement of the right hemisphere has been mentioned frequently in the literature. We have found left-handedness in the family of right-handed patients who had dysphasia with involvement of the left hemisphere, and we doubt that there is any significant difference in the two groups. Similarly, right-handedness occurs in the family of left-handed patients who have had dysphasia with involvement of either hemisphere, and again we doubt that there is any significant difference in the two groups. Kennedy's (1916) suggestion regarding "stock brainedness" has not been substantiated. Recently, Subirana (1956) has maintained that the occurrence of left-handedness in the family of the right-handed may explain the transient rather than the persistent dysphasia with vascular lesions of the left half. Recovery from aphasia can occur, depending on many factors —particularly the size and locus of the lesion. The significance of familial sinistrality in Subirana's patients (particularly regarding the children of the patients) is not clear in our present stage of knowledge.

In the right-handed less than one per cent have some representation of speech in the right hemisphere, according to our data. Subirana (1956) reported 5.9% of right-handed patients with transient dysphasia and persistent left hemiplegia, thus indicating some speech representation on the right. This percentage is probably too high for the "normal right-handed population," as the patients were selected on the basis of persistent left hemiplegia and/or aphasia. Other reports in the literature can be criticized in a similar manner. It is believed that less than one per cent of the right-handed have some representation of speech on the right.

Is all of speech represented on the right in these right-handed? We do not know. But there are enough cases reported with persistent dysphasia and only right hemispheral involvement to state that sometimes all of speech is represented on the right in right-handers. In others there may be bilateral representation, but this is not proved.

Less than ten per cent of the left-handed have some, and probably all, speech representation on the right according to our data. Now this is not the type of data one would expect from animal experimentation, as we cannot prove the other left-handed—93.3%—would not have shown dysphasia were the whole right hemisphere removed. However, the comparison of the percentage of left-handers showing dysphasia after operation on the left (72.2%) and the right hemisphere (6.7%) is the significant factor. It is even more significant because the speech areas were more often encroached upon in the right hemisphere than in the left. Thus, if it were true that the representation of speech in the left-handed is usually on the right or bilateral (Goodglass and Quadfasel, 1954), our percentages for transient dysphasia would be quite different.

Again, there is no comparable series of patients in the literature. Adding our cases to those in the literature, there are 144 left-handers with dysphasia—55% involving the left hemisphere and 45% involving the right. And there are one and one-half times as many negative cases (left-handers without dysphasia) involving the right hemisphere (33) as the left (21). Summarizing the literature in this manner yields a confusing picture. Presented with a left-hander who has aphasia, "my bookie quotes odds of 9 to 1 that the lesion is in the left half and 1 to 11 that it is in the right!"

Is all of speech in the left or right half in a particular left-

hander? Once again we do not know. In some it is certainly unilateral, as persistent dysphasia has been reported with involvement
of either hemisphere—more often the left. A definite possibility of
bilateral representation of speech exists. If bilaterality occurs, our
figures could be interpreted as indicating it to be more frequent
in the left-handed.*

The sodium amytal aphasia test (see Chapter V, page 86) has
not given clear-cut evidence of bilateral representation of speech
but has shown some equivocal results.

The type of disturbance in speech which occurs with disease of
the right hemisphere seems different in most instances from that
with disease of the left. Permanent aphasia rarely if ever occurs
with involvement of *only* the right half. Head's (1926) single case
had "semantic aphasia;" this type is quite different from other
aphasias and might be considered a disturbance of some other
psychological process and not a dysphasia at all.† Schiller's (1947)
two patients had, as their only residual defect, difficulty in learning
to write with the right hand, which, he stated, was much more
marked than in other patients learning to write with the left hand.
Perhaps they were left-handed because of original minimal clumsi-
ness of the right hand.

Bucy (1951) remarks that transient aphasia may follow operation involving the cerebellar fossa. We have seen a similar case.
Perhaps the right hemisphere has no more to do with speech than
the cerebellum in the normal person.

2. *On handedness*

Bouillaud (1825, 1865) had contended that the faculty of speech
was localized in the frontal lobes. In order to explain the absence
of aphasia with disease on the right, handedness was introduced.
None of the anthropoids or lower animals, as a species, speak or
use one extremity predominantly, though individual animals may
prefer to use one limb. For centuries philosophers have pointed

---

* One must remember that even though dysphasia was thirteen times more frequent in the left-handed with right hemispheral involvement, the difference is not
statistically significant.

† Since 1926 others have used the adjective "semantic" in modifying aphasia to
refer to different disorders, and they have stated that semantic difficulties occur in
all dysphasics; this is not true if we adhere to Head's definition (see Chapter IV,
page 67).

out that in addition to speaking, man is usually right-handed. Thus, Bouillaud's and Broca's theory seemed a logical one.

Sir Russell Brain has called attention to the incidence of left-handedness in biblical times. In the year 1406 B.C., there were seven hundred chosen left-handed men who "could sling stones at an hair breadth, and not miss." Thus, 3.7 per cent of the army of the children of Benjamin were chosen left-handers (Judges, 20). In modern times, the left-handed have been estimated at between 1 and 30 per cent of the population; the higher frequencies have occurred in mental hospitals, where there is a higher frequency of brain disease. In 1951, Rife stated that there were between 10 and 15 million left-handed people in the United States (6.7–10% of the population).

What determines handedness? One factor has been noted, namely: a cerebral injury may produce hemiplegia and necessitate the use of the opposite hand. All people with weakness of one hand from cerebral disease do not use the other hand predominantly, but certainly most do, and some that do not have bilateral brain disease.

Subirana et al. (1952) found more abnormal brain waves in the left-handed than in the right-handed among 316 normal children. Schiller (1947) noted that his left-handed patients had greater difficulty learning to write with the right hand than the right-handed did in learning to use the left hand after cerebral injury. These two observations may indicate that, in the absence of weakness of the right hand, brain disease sometimes may determine left-handedness.

Weakness of one upper extremity from other causes than cerebral disease also will determine the preferred hand.

Blau (1946) suggested that negativism was the cause of left-handedness. Negativism may be compared with the mutism observed in autistic children. Psychiatric causes may determine left-handedness in some individuals.

Studies on handedness in relation to Mendelian laws usually have not taken into consideration the previously mentioned factors for determining handedness. Rife (1951) stated that 50% of the children were left-handed when both parents were left-handed, 16.7% of the children were left-handed when one parent was left-handed, and 6.3% of the children were left-handed when neither parent was left-handed. He pointed out that such percentages may be due either to heredity or to environment.

Pooled data from several investigators show that in identical twins 78% of the pairs are right-handed, 2% are left-handed, and 20% have one right- and one left-handed—"an almost perfect random distribution in which approximately 12 per cent of the individuals are left-handed" (Rife, 1951). It has been suggested that this relation could be explained on mirror-imaging. Rife (1951) pointed out that there has been no correlation between different traits with respect to mirror-imaging, as would be expected if mirror-imaging depended solely upon how early the embryo divided.

Rife (1941) found no significant relationship between handedness and sex. Rife and Kloepfer (1943) found no significant relationship between handedness and blood groups. Rife (1951) found dermatoglyphics to be related to handedness. For example, patterns in the form of loops and whorls may be present in the thenar (first interdigital) area (T/I). Ten per cent of 3,721 right-handers have T/I patterns, and 14 per cent of 1,536 left-handers have T/I patterns. Rife concludes on the basis of this and similar differences in other palm patterns that handedness "cannot be due solely to postnatal environmental circumstances." However, these differences in percentage are not impressive.

In the genetic literature no better evidence could be found that handedness is inherited according to Mendelian laws.

3. *On shift of dominance*

We have discussed handedness and the occurrence of aphasia in relation to handedness. Now let us consider the so-called shift of dominance. From the time of Broca, much has been written on the recovery of speech, even though a lesion was found at autopsy in one of the so-called speech areas. It has been assumed that the homologous area of the other hemisphere took over the function of the diseased part.

According to this theory, one aspect of speech, such as comprehension of spoken words, might be shifted to the opposite side; whereas, the other aspects of speech would remain on the original side. There are no cases in the literature with a second lesion on the opposite side and aphasia. Cases such as that of Barlow (1877) show evidence of pseudobulbar palsy.

Twenty-four of our patients are known to have had aphasia with injury occurring after the age of two years. Sixteen of these twenty-four again had aphasia after operation for control of seizures. And, for example, if the lesion and excision were in the temporo-parietal region, the patient might have disturbances in the visual and auditory components of speech on both occasions.

Objection could be made that the entire area had not been destroyed. However, the lesions and subsequent cortical excisions are comparable in size to those reported in the literature. It is not contended that permanent aphasia would result necessarily from removal of the entire left hemisphere. As Krynauw (1950) and others have shown, a complete removal of a hemisphere diseased from early life may be carried out without disturbance in speech. Hillier (1954) reported return of speech following excision of the left hemisphere subsequent to two subtotal removals of a glioma in a teenager. Also, the patient of Zollinger (1935) had some return of speech before death three weeks after a hemispherectomy in an adult.

It is contended that aphasia usually results after a second or even a third operation on the left hemisphere for control of seizures when the lesion is small relative to the whole hemisphere.

There is no proof that the opposite hemisphere may become "dominant" for one component of speech, though this remains a theoretical possibility. It is our opinion that when there is a lesion sufficiently large to cause transfer, that transfer is for all components of speech.

D. *Summary*

The presence or absence of aphasia has been determined for 522 patients upon whom operation was performed for treatment of focal cerebral seizures. The handedness was classed as right-, left-, predominantly right-, and predominantly left-handed; all of our so-called ambidextrous patients preferred to use one specific hand for the majority of things. In the final analysis there was no difference between the left- and predominantly left-handed, or between the right- and predominantly right-handed, and they have been grouped together as left- or right-handed.

With exclusion of cases with cerebral injury prior to the age of two years, there is no difference in the frequency of aphasia after operation on the left hemisphere between the left- and right-handed.

With similar exclusion there is no significant difference in the frequency of aphasia after operation on the right hemisphere between the right- and left-handed. Dysphasia is, of course, quite rare with involvement of only the right hemisphere.

This conclusion is at variance with most of the opinions in the literature. In almost one hundred years, only about 140 cases have been reported with aphasia and involvement of only the right hemisphere. It seems clear that the left hemisphere is usually dominant for speech, regardless of handedness. The reason why the right hemisphere is sometimes dominant for speech remains unclear, but it is not related solely to handedness.

Handedness is determined by multiple factors including pathological, psychological (normal and abnormal), hereditary, and perhaps, unknown factors. Man seems to have acquired language and to have become right-handed at about the same time in evolution. Perhaps the reason man is right-handed is one of pure chance—then: custom and laziness. The representation of speech in the left hemisphere is due to a simplicity of function for the brain. Brain function and handedness may be unrelated except by disease.

Because recovery of speech occurs following damage of part of the left hemisphere, it does not indicate that the right hemisphere usually takes over the function of the homologous area on the left. Aphasia usually occurs after a second injury to the left half. It seems that if other areas on the left are capable of functioning during speech, they will. After complete removal of the left hemisphere, then the right half is used. If this occurs early in life, speech develops or returns much more readily than if it occurs in adulthood. An abnormally functioning brain may prevent regression of the aphasia, as shown by one of our patients who improved after operation and control of his seizures with no evidence of remaining abnormally functioning brain.

CHAPTER VII

MAPPING THE SPEECH AREA

W. P.

∿∿∿∿∿∿∿∿∿∿∿∿∿∿∿∿∿∿∿∿∿∿∿

∿∿∿∿∿∿∿∿∿∿∿∿∿∿∿∿∿∿∿∿∿∿∿

A. *Forbidden territory*

TWENTY-FIVE years ago we were embarking on the treatment of focal epilepsy by radical surgical excision of abnormal areas of brain (Foerster and Penfield, 1930a and 1930b; Penfield, 1930). In the beginning it was our practice to refuse radical operation upon the dominant hemisphere unless a lesion lay anteriorly in the frontal lobe or posteriorly in the occipital lobe. Like other neurosurgeons, we feared that removal of cortex in other parts of this hemisphere would produce aphasia. The left temporal lobe and the fronto-centro-parietal areas were considered to be devoted to mechanisms of speech, and aphasia literature gave no clear guide as to just what might and what might not be removed with impunity.

But patients continued to present themselves in increasing numbers with focal epilepsy that had followed scars and atrophic lesions and small tumors, placed by chance within this general area. Many of these patients were not aphasic. Some had not been aphasic at the time of a well localized previous injury. And so we were emboldened gradually to make more and more excisions within this forbidden territory.

During this period of exploration we developed a method of *mapping the speech cortex* by using electrical interference on the surface of the cortex at the time of operation. This will be described in detail below. This was most important to us during the earlier stages of exploration, and it has provided us with a most important body of information for this monograph.

But curiously enough, now that we have carried out the test some hundreds of times, we find it necessary to use it much less frequently. This is because of the growing ability to predict speech area limits, and because recent employment of the *amytal aphasia test* (Chapter V) carried out before operation can now answer that most important question as to which hemisphere contains the speech areas.

The amytal test is particularly useful when there has been a lesion or an injury, early in life, to the left hemisphere, especially one that caused the patient to change from right-handedness to left-handedness. In such a case, wide excision may be necessary for cure, but the surgeon must know for certain whether or not speech has been displaced to the right.

The cortical excisions, carried out with increasing temerity after operative exploration and while the patient continued to talk, served the purposes of treatment of focal epileptic seizures. They did not destroy the patient's ability to speak, although aphasia frequently appeared as a reaction following operation, to disappear again when convalescence was over.

Thus, two major sources of new information have become available: 1) the excisions of cortex about speech areas, and 2) mapping of the speech areas themselves by the electrical interfering-stimulation during operation. The aphasia appearing during an epileptic seizure and the transient aphasia that follows operation are minor sources of information. The purpose of this monograph is to summarize and to study this new information. Conclusions will appear in later chapters. This chapter will be devoted largely to identification of cortical speech areas during operation and to aphasia as it appears during focal epileptic seizures.

B. *Preoperative study*

In cases of focal cerebral seizures, the epileptogenic lesion most often proves to be an atrophic area of cortex. Its location can usually be determined by careful study of the pattern of the patient's habitual seizures. *Epileptic aphasia* occurs when the seizure discharge involves the speech areas of the dominant hemisphere during a partial attack. The pattern of the attack must be studied from the beginning so as to discover whether aphasia is present as an initial phenomenon or later, during the evolution of the patient's seizures. This can be established by a critical observer during his minor attacks. But unless attacks are frequent, it may be necessary to induce a seizure slowly by administration of metrazol while an electroencephalogram is being run.

If aphasia seems to be the initial phenomenon in a seizure, it is still necessary to determine whether epileptic discharge begins in an adjacent silent area or in the speech area itself. If it is clear that epileptic discharge begins in a speech area, operation is better not undertaken at all. Excision within the major temporo-parietal speech area is not to be considered. But excision of superior parietal or anterior temporal areas is now clearly justifiable.

Preoperative electroencephalograms are of the greatest assistance in localization. But when the focus is in the region of the Sylvian fissure of the dominant hemisphere, it may be difficult or impossible to judge from that test whether discharge begins in a speech area or not. If the focal discharge is most active in an electrode placed in the pharynx (pharyngeal lead), which is often the case in temporal lobe epilepsy, one may be relatively secure in the belief that the discharge begins in the hippocampal zone. We shall show below that this portion of the temporal lobe plays no role in the mechanism of speech.

Preoperative decision as to which hemisphere is dominant for speech has already been discussed in Chapter V. The amytal test which is invaluable in doubtful cases was described there.

C. *Procedures in the operating room*

In the treatment of focal epilepsy caused by an atrophic lesion of the cortex the operation of *osteoplastic craniotomy* is best carried out under local anaesthesia, especially when the dominant hemisphere is to be exposed. It is essential, therefore, that there be sympathetic understanding between patient and surgeon. Before the procedure of *speech mapping* can be described, the organization of the operating room must be visualized (Fig. VII-1).

Patient and surgeon are separated by a tent made of the surgical

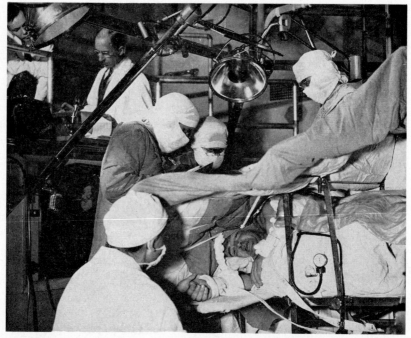

FIG. VII-1. Layout of operating room. The surgeon is filling in a sketch of the brain. In the background Dr. Jasper is seen recording an electrocortico-gram behind the glass partition of the observing stand, while his associate, Dr. Guy Courtois, watches. The patient is seen fully conscious and comfort-able, thanks to local analgesia, with the anesthetist, Dr. André Pasquet, who is acting as observer, beside him. Beyond the observer is the square window through which the photographs of the brain are taken by means of the mirror placed above the table.

"drapes." They cannot see each other, but they must be able to talk back and forth. During the time of electrical stimulation of the cortex, there is need of a third person, an observer, who sits with the patient under the tent. The anaesthetist,* who is never very far away, often undertakes this added service.

Although the operation is begun under local analgesia, it is completed under general anaesthesia. This method is better called combined regional and general anaesthesia (Penfield and Pasquet, 1954). The cooperation and guidance of the anaesthetist is most important to the surgeon from the beginning.

* Over the years we have been helped greatly by the anaesthetists in charge, es-pecially Miss Mary Roach, R.N., Dr. André Pasquet, and Professor Richard Gilbert.

1. *Stimulator and stimulating electrode*

Three types of stimulator have been employed at different times in the study of the cases to be reported here: a) thyratron stimulator, b) Rahm stimulator, and c) square wave generator.*

The Rahm stimulator has been used in the majority of cases reported here. But in every case the minimum or threshold strength of stimulus was determined by gradually increasing the voltage until a sensory response was obtained from the postcentral gyrus. It was often necessary to increase that slightly to produce movement from the precentral gyrus. Response from the supplementary motor area might be obtained with the same voltage or after a minor increase. Responses from the auditory and visual areas of temporal and occipital lobes usually called for double the threshold voltage required on the postcentral gyrus; and for the localization of speech areas of the cortex, the voltage was likewise usually set at double the threshold intensity. That is, if 2 volts were the minimum required to produce somatic sensation on the postcentral gyrus with the square wave generator (set at 2 milliseconds and 60 cycles), then the voltage was raised to 3 or 4 volts for speech testing.

Either bipolar or unipolar electrodes may be used for stimulation. It was our practice to use a bipolar electrode until 1951. Since that time we have used a unipolar electrode, coated except at the tip, so that it may be passed into the brain and stimulation carried out deep to its convexity when desired.

2. *Routine of cortical mapping*

It has come to be our practice, as a preliminary to excision of epileptogenic areas, to map out functional areas of the cortex by stimulation. This is made possible by the help of a conscious and cooperative patient. Mapping makes the cortical excision safer and more exact. It also produces at times the initial phenomenon in

---

* The thyratron, as employed in physiological laboratories, was used before 1945. After July 1945, a modified Rahm stimulator was used, which provided a "saw tooth" wave form that varied in duration with the frequency of stimulation. The frequency used was usually 60, sometimes varied down to 30 per second. Since March 2nd, 1951, a square wave generator built under the direction of Dr. Herbert Jasper has been used. It produces rectangular unidirectional pulses between 0.2 and 5 milliseconds in duration. Frequency and peak-voltage are controlled.

the patient's habitual seizure and so helps the surgeon to lay his plans for curative excision. When a positive effect has been produced, a small ticket bearing a number is dropped on the surface of the brain, and the nature of the effect or response is dictated by the surgeon to a secretary who sits in the viewing stand behind a glass partition. Thus the motor, sensory, and psychical responses become a part of the operative record, and any unusual or doubtful responses can be verified by repeated stimulation without warning the patient. These matters have been described and discussed elsewhere (Penfield and Rasmussen, 1950; Penfield and Jasper, 1954).

The records of these operations that will be used in this study consist of the dictated account referred to above, photographs of the brain before removal of the tickets, and a drawing made by the operator (with sterile materials) during the procedure, which records his understanding of the exact position of stimulation points and the extent and position of any cortical excision that may be carried out.

3. *Activation and arrest*

The invariable effect of simple electrical stimulation in any area of cortex is to produce interference with the normal employment of that area. In some areas the stimulus produces activation as well. In other areas this seems to be impossible and only interference is produced. Take several examples:

If the electric current is applied to the Rolandic motor area or the supplementary motor area (Fig. II-10), the result may be a movement which the patient cannot resist by any exercise of his will. Or it often happens that there is simple inhibition of specific movements, and the arm or leg lies motionless, even though the patient tries voluntarily to move it. In either case he cannot utilize the area of cortex for his own purposes during stimulation.

Stimulation of the postcentral gyrus may produce, for example, a sensation of tingling in the contralateral thumb. During the application of the electrode, the patient cannot use the thumb for exploring the texture of external objects because it is numb.

Stimulation of the gray matter within the calcarine fissure of the left occipital lobe may cause the patient to see simple colored figures to the right of him, but for the moment, he is wholly or partly blind to the right. He cannot employ the stimulated zone of cortex for its normal visual function.

And so it is with those areas in the cerebral cortex that are normally employed for speech. Application of an electrical current to one of them produces local interference or aphasic arrest. Thus, the man cannot for the moment use the area. There is no positive response to the stimulation. No movement is produced and no sensation. No positive psychical process is set in motion. The stimulation does not summon words to the mind of the man nor does it cause him to speak.

If he is lying quietly on the operating table, he has no means of knowing that the electrode has been applied to a speech area in his own dominant hemisphere. But if, at the moment of stimulation, the patient is trying to talk, he discovers, to his astonishment, that he is aphasic. He may use some words but he cannot find others. Or, on the other hand, he may be speechless, though he tries to speak and perhaps snaps his fingers in exasperation. After withdrawal of the electrode, words may come with a rush, and he explains what he had been trying to say but could not.

D. *Exploration of speech territory*

A technique of speech-area mapping was elaborated and put to practical use (by W. P. in 1945-46) with the help of our associate, Dr. Preston Robb, who acted as observer in the operating theatre and studied the patients before and after operation (Robb, 1946). The procedure has been elaborated further since then, until at present the localization of these areas can be carried out rapidly without the loss of more than ten or fifteen minutes of operating time. *Speech mapping* is carried out as follows: Recording electrodes are applied to the cortex for the usual routine study of the nature and position of electrographic abnormalities of the epileptic type. When that is finished, the recording electrodes are left in place while speech mapping is carried out. A stimulating electrode is then applied here and there to establish the limits of cortex that are essential to normal speech. It was pointed out above that in the speech areas, stimulation produces only local functional interference.

NAMING. The observer sits close to the patient where he can

see and be seen (Fig. VII-1), and patient and observer can talk easily. The observer presents to the patient a succession of card pictures, and the latter is requested to respond to each by saying, for example, "That is a ship," "That is a dog," and so on.

The operator, listening to this simple exercise, applies his electrode to the cortex at one point and then another in the area he wishes to explore. If the naming continues without interruption, a minute square of paper is dropped on the brain at the point of application of the electrode to show that the result was negative.

When interference with the patient's speech is produced, a numbered ticket is placed at the point of application, and then, after discussion with the observer, the operator dictates the character of this speech interference.

COUNTING. The patient is asked to count, and while he is doing so, the operator applies his stimulating electrode to selected areas of cortex. He listens to any change that may appear in the progress of the counting at the time of application and notes what happens when the electrode is withdrawn. This procedure of counting is particularly useful for observation of induced dysarthria, of complete speech arrest, and of vocalization.

WRITING. The observer arranges paper and pencil so that the patient can reply to questions or name the cards and the objects shown him by writing down the answer. The operator then applies the electrode to appropriate points while listening to the conversation of observer and patient.

READING. Similar determinations are carried out while the patient reads aloud.

During all of these tests (naming, counting, writing, reading), neither observer nor patient is aware of the time or location of electrode application. The observer, however, has the advantage of being able to see the patient, so that he and the operator should consult after each positive electrode effect.

The "reading test" and the "writing test" have not been used enough for the results to be statistically significant. The "naming test" has been useful in demonstrating whether or not the arrest of speech or the interference with speech is dysphasic (aphasic) in character.*

---

* The terms aphasia and dysphasia are defined elsewhere. They are used here

Before assuming that a convolution, on which electrode application has produced *aphasic arrest*, is really to be considered part of a cortical speech-area, we have taken great care to be sure that the stimulation has not produced epileptic after-discharge. This may inactivate neighboring convolutions. Confusion on this score may be avoided, also, by noting the time of appearance of aphasic arrest following application of the electrode to the cortex and the duration after withdrawal. But the use of electrocorticography during speech mapping adds greater certainty.

If a small electrographic seizure follows stimulation, the result is informative, but no localizing value is given to the trial. The strength of the stimulus is usually reduced before proceeding.*

Positive results, when properly controlled, are of real value for the purposes of the operation and from the point of view of anatomical study. But negative results of stimulation must not be accepted as clear evidence that the area in question is not related to speech. If stimulation at the same voltage produces aphasic arrest in one area, then the negative results are obviously more significant in neighboring areas. When stimulation produces aphasic arrest, it is clear that the hemisphere exposed is dominant for speech, for we have never been able to produce such an effect from the non-dominant hemisphere.

The following case of focal cerebral seizures, due to an atrophic lesion of the cortex, will be reported in some detail as an example of *cortical exploration, speech mapping,* and *temporal lobectomy* (partial) in the dominant hemisphere.

E. *Case Example*

This man, C. H., aged thirty-seven and right-handed, received a blow on the right vertex of the skull while serving in the Canadian Merchant Marine. Attacks began three months later and continued for six years, in spite of medication, up to the time of his operation in 1948.

Minor attacks, as described by his wife who was a former nurse,

---

interchangeably to describe interference with the ideational processes of speech, in contrast to motor difficulties of articulation called anarthria or dysarthria.

* Our associate, Herbert Jasper, has controlled these tests by electrocorticography, helping us to perfect this method, as he has in many other projects that call for neurophysiological insight.

were as follows: He would seem to turn pale and his pupils would dilate. At the same time, he was confused and might swallow or say things that seemed to have no relation to the present, such as, "It is caught," or, "It shows."

Later, he would have no recollection of such seizures and there was no warning aura. During the attack he would act in an automatic manner, continuing to drive an automobile or to walk.

Major attacks began in the same way, but there was turning of head and eyes to the right followed by blinking of the eyelids and generalized convulsive movements. Aphasia had never been observed following the attacks.

Dr. Donald McRae reported that pneumoencephalography showed moderate enlargement of the tip of the left temporal horn of the lateral ventrical.

Dr. Jasper reported that the pre-operative electroencephalograms showed random "spike and sharp wave" abnormalities originating on the under surface of the left temporal lobe (foramen ovale lead).

The pattern of attacks, the electrogram, and the pneumoencephalogram all pointed to the anterior portion of the left temporal lobe. It was concluded that the source of the seizures and the focus of electrographic abnormality were in the anterior and mesial portion of that lobe. It seemed likely that the blow on the head had produced a "contre coup" injury there.

The attacks were classified as focal cerebral seizures characterized by automatism. Operative cortical excision was recommended.

Craniotomy. An osteoplastic opening was made in the temporal region, a bone flap being turned down on the attachment of the temporal muscle, and the dura opened (Fig. VII-2). A few adhesions were found between dura and temporal pole, and there was whitening of the arachnoid over the fissure of Sylvius anteriorly (Fig. II-3), and evidence of severe bruising of the anterior tip of the lobe (see Frontispiece).

Electrocorticography was carried out, the recording electrodes being placed directly on the brain. A focus of high-voltage sharp waves was found to be present on the under surface of the anterior end of the lobe.

Electrical stimulation was carried out while the electrocorticograph continued to record. A threshold strength of stimulus (60

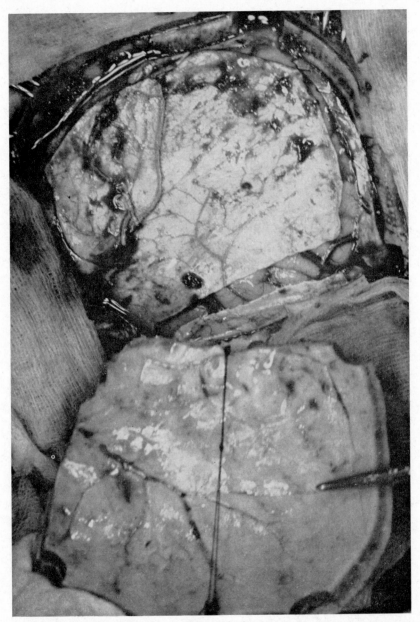

F‍ig. VII-2. CASE C. H. Left craniotomy. The osteoplastic bone-flap has been turned down, and the underlying dura mater has been cut so that the brain may be exposed.

cycles, 1 volt) was used at the beginning. The order of stimulations is indicated by the numbers on the tickets that have been dropped on the cortex (Fig. VII-3). A few of the patient's responses may

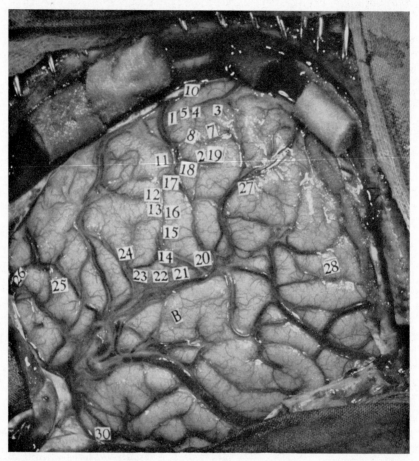

Fig. VII-3. CASE C. H. The dura has been turned back to expose the cortex. The left temporal lobe is seen below the fissure of Sylvius. Compare with Fig. VII-5 and with the Frontispiece. The numbered tickets, dropped on the surface of the cortex, indicate points of positive response to electrical stimulation. See text for explanation.

be given here just as they were dictated during operation. Position of the points referred to is shown by the position of the numbered tickets in Figures VII-3, VII-4, and VII-5.

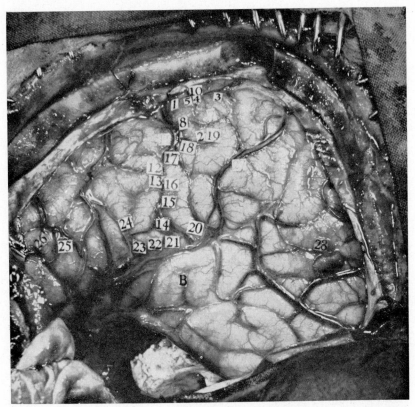

Fig. VII-4. CASE C. H. The anterior temporal lobe has been removed, exposing white matter of the temporal stem. The insula is in shadow above the stem.

POSTCENTRAL GYRUS

1—Tingling right thumb and slight movement.

19—Sensation in lower lip, outside.

17—Sensation right upper lip, inside.

16—Tingling in right side of tongue at the tip.

14—Sensation in the "joint of the jaw and in the lower lip, inside."

PRECENTRAL GYRUS

11—"Feeling in my throat which stopped my speech."

12—Quivering of jaw in a "sidewise manner."

13—Pulling of jaw to right.

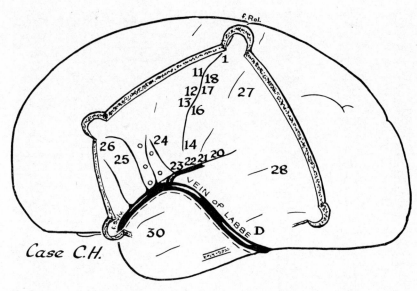

Fɪɢ. VII-5. CASE C. H. Drawing of operation. Broken line indicates the extent of left temporal lobe removal. Aphasia (aphasic arrest) was produced by stimulating electrode placed at points 26, 27, and 28. Anarthria (motor speech arrest) was produced at points 23 and 24. Strength of current used for points 20-26 was 2 volts; increased to 3 volts for 27 and 28.

LOWER ROLANDIC

20—Jaw pulled up, and there was tingling in it—not more on one side than on the other.

21—Opening of jaw.

22—Tongue seemed to move and there was tingling inside of lower lip.

Speech arrest due to motor effect.

23—Stimulation carried out while the patient was talking. He stopped but vocalized a little. After cessation of stimulation, he said he had been unable to speak.

23—Repeated when patient was not trying to talk. There was no vocalization and he observed nothing.

24—Patient tried to talk and mouth moved to the right, but he made no sound.

SPEECH-MAPPING—APHASIC ARREST

25—The patient hesitated and then named "butterfly" correctly. Stimulation was carried out then below this point and at a number of points on the two narrow gyri that separate 25 from 24, but the result was negative—no interference with the naming process. The points of negative stimulation are shown by the small circles in Figure VII-5.

26—The patient said, "Oh, I know what it is. That is what you put in your shoes." After withdrawal of the electrode he said, "foot."

27—Unable to name tree which was being shown to him. Instead he said, "I know what it is." Electrode was withdrawn then and he said, "tree."

28—The patient became unable to name as soon as the electrode was placed here. When asked why he did not name the picture shown, he said, "no." He continued to be silent after withdrawal of the stimulating electrode.

Dr. Jasper reported that the electrograph showed afterdischarge which began in a nearby recording electrode and spread to involve the whole temporal region. During this, the patient continued to be unable to name and no longer would answer anything.

The electrographic seizure stopped suddenly and the patient spoke at once. "Now I can talk," he said. "Butterfly." Dr. Pasquet, who was acting as observer, had concluded from the patient's expression and movements that he had been trying to answer all through the stimulation and during the after-discharge.

When he began to talk he was asked why he had not been able to name the picture, and he replied, "I couldn't get that word 'butterfly' and then I tried to get the word 'moth.'"

30—Patient tried to talk but could not. The stimulation was followed by after-discharge at six per second, recorded on the posterior and inferior temporal lobe. After the attack was over he said, "I tried to answer and couldn't."

The results of stimulation at points 28 and 30 should be given no exact localizing value. The temporal cortex gave after-discharge to the two-volt stimulus at each point, although there had been none when parietal and frontal cortices were stimulated with the same electric current.

Surgical removal. Excision of the anterior portion of the temporal lobe was carried out by suction along the line of fissure marked by the vein of Labbé (Fig. VII-5). A traumatic scar associated with dense gliosis was found on the under surface of the temporal lobe anteriorly. The patient has not been completely cured by operation.

There was no evidence of aphasia until twenty hours after operation. Following that, there was progressive development of profound aphasia. This began to improve at the end of two weeks and cleared up finally several weeks later.

Postoperative aphasia developing several days after operation is due to a condition called *neuroparalytic edema*. It develops, usually, on the second or third day and reaches its height on the fifth to the tenth day. Then it recedes. It seems to be due to exposure of adjacent brain to the air and to post-operative changes in circulation.

CHAPTER VIII

THE EVIDENCE FROM CORTICAL MAPPING

ℒ. ℛ.

~~~~~~

A. Alterations in speech from
    electrical interference
B. Handedness and dominance
C. Discussion
D. Summary

~~~~~~

A. *Alterations in speech from electrical interference*

THE brain is exposed by means of a large craniotomy, with the patient under local anesthesia. The patient is asked to count or to name a series of pictures of objects. The electrode is placed at various cortical points while this counting or naming is occurring, as outlined in Chapter VII. These results are now summarized.

Jefferson (1935) reported inability to speak during and after stimulation of the angular gyrus, but he did not use this test as a means of mapping out the extent of the speech areas of the cortex. Foerster (1936) noted grunts and groans during stimulation of the lower Rolandic region. In 1935, Penfield was surprised to hear a clear, sustained vowel cry upon stimulation of the precentral gyrus. This and other cases were reported in 1938.

Brickner (1940), as a witness at operation, noted repetition of words and syllables from stimulation of what Penfield has called the supplementary motor area. This has been confirmed by Penfield and Welch (1951), and Erickson and Woolsey (1951). Other reports on the effects of stimulation have been made on the series of patients presented in this monograph by Robb (1948), Penfield and Rasmussen (1949, 1950), and Roberts (1949, 1951, 1952, 1958a, 1958b), and these will not be reviewed.

As noted in the previous chapter, while the patient is naming pictures of objects, the electric current is applied to various cortical areas. The results of this naming test are here summarized. The electrical current instead of stimulating may interfere with or arrest function; for this reason we have used the terms "electrical arrest" and "electrical interference" in referring to negative effects, rather than "electrical stimulation."

Stimulation has produced two effects on speech: 1) positive or vocalization, and 2) negative or inability to vocalize or to use words properly. No intelligible word has been induced while the patient is silent. Vocalization is a sustained or interrupted vowel cry, which at times may have a consonant component. It is produced by stimulation of the motor areas called Rolandic and supplementary by Penfield and Rasmussen (1950) (Figs. VIII-1 and VIII-2). For

VOCALIZATION

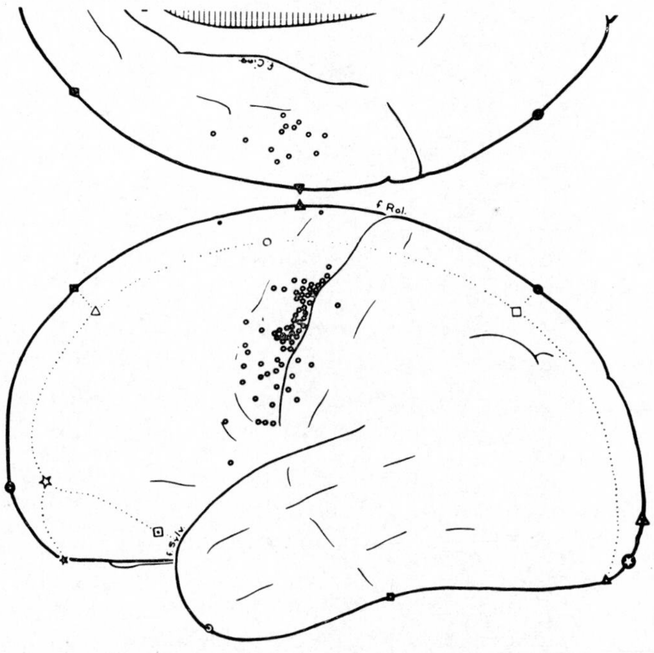

FIG. VIII-1. Vocalization, which is a sustained or interrupted vowel cry, has been produced by stimulation at these points in the left hemisphere.

vocalization the Rolandic area includes the precentral and post-central gyri for lips, jaw, and tongue; the supplementary area includes the superior and medial aspects of the intermediate precentral region of Campbell (1905). Vocalization occurs during stimulation of either dominant or non-dominant motor areas.

Electrical interference involving the left hemisphere has produced interference with speech at the points shown in Figure VIII-3. We believe that some of the stimulations of the Rolandic region and the supplementary motor area are interfering with the motor control of speech organs, as they may be accompanied by movements of the face and tongue.

VOCALIZATION

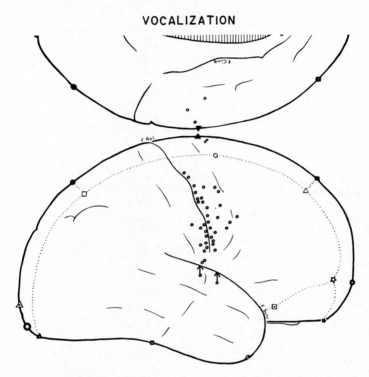

FIG. VIII-2. Vocalization has occurred during stimulation at these points in the right hemisphere.

These negative effects of electrical interference are classified, arbitrarily, into various types of response. Total arrest of speech or inability to vocalize spontaneously—the first effect—occurs not only in the motor areas, but outside of them (Fig. VIII-4).

The second effect is hesitation and slurring of speech (Fig. VIII-5). The third and fourth effects are distortion and repetition of words and syllables, grouped together in Figure VIII-6. Distortion differs from slurring in that the distorted sound is not a word but an unintelligible sound. The unintelligible sound has been repeated. Repetition of numbers while counting and repetition of other words and syllables have occurred.

Antedating the use of the naming test, the patient was asked to

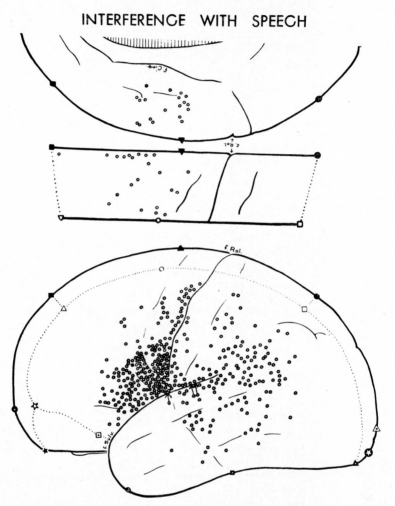

INTERFERENCE WITH SPEECH

Fig. VIII-3. Electrical interference has produced interference with speech at these points in the left hemisphere. When the electric current has been applied to other areas, such as the frontal pole or the occipital lobe, no difficulty in speech has been noted. The types of disturbance are given in subsequent figures.

count while the electric current was applied to the cortex. The fifth effect is confusion of numbers while counting (Fig. VIII-7).

This confusion is illustrated by the patient jumping from "six" to "twenty" and then back to "nine." He continued counting correctly after withdrawal of the electrode. Words other than numbers were not used, i.e. he had the proper "set" but was unable to give the correct numbers.

ARREST OF SPEECH

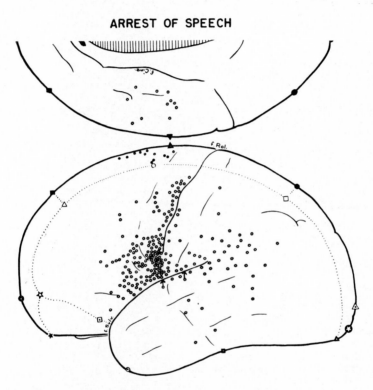

Fig. VIII-4. Complete arrest of speech occurred during electrical arrest at these points. We believe that those results in the motor areas are due to an interference with motor mechanisms, whereas those outside of motor areas are due to an interference with speech mechanisms.

Inability to name with retained ability to speak is the sixth effect (Fig. VIII-8). An example is, "That is a . . . I know. That is a . . ." When the current was removed, the patient named the picture correctly. Another example is, "Oh, I know what it is. That is what you put in your shoes." After withdrawal of the stimulating electrodes, the patient immediately said "foot." Still another example is inability to name a comb. When asked its use, he said, "I comb my hair." When asked again to name it, he couldn't until the electrode was removed.

Misnaming with evidence of perseveration (Fig. VIII-9) occurs when the patient names a "butterfly" as the stimulating electrode is applied, then calls a table a "butterfly;" after the current is removed, he names the picture correctly. At other times the "per-

HESITATION AND SLURRING OF SPEECH

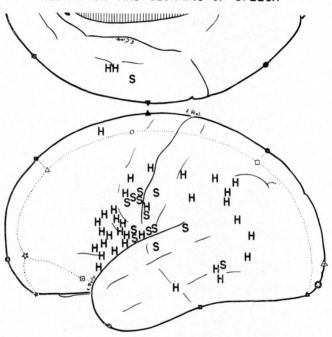

Fig. VIII-5. Hesitation and slurring of speech occurred when the electrode was applied to these points.

severated word" has been a correct word used not just before the electrode was applied, but perhaps a minute or two before.

The eighth type of response is the most unusual (Fig. VIII-10). In misnaming without perseveration, the patient may use words somewhat closely related in sound, such as "camel" for "comb." Or he may use a synonym, such as "cutters" for "scissors," "hay" for "bed," and "moth" for "butterfly." Or an entirely unrelated word, such as "rink" for "scissors," or "cone" for "hammer," has been used.

The electric current has been applied to the cortex while the patient was reading or writing. The number of such tests has been too few for general conclusions. It may be stated, however, that alterations in reading and writing have occurred when the elec-

DISTORTION AND REPETITION OF WORDS AND SYLLABLES

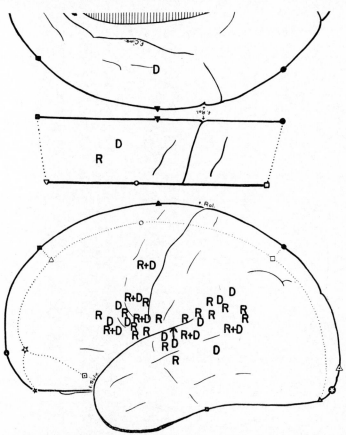

FIG. VIII-6. Distortion and repetition of words and syllables was noted when the electrode was placed at these points. Distortion differs from slurring in that the distorted sound is unrecognizable as a word.

trode has been applied to anterior and superior as well as posterior speech areas.

The location of the points of electrical interference of the left hemisphere producing the eight different types of response are seen in the various figures. The last six types are classified as aphasic types of response in Figure VIII-11. These responses—distortion and repetition of words, confusion of numbers while counting, inability to name with retained ability to speak, and misnaming with or without perseveration—are obtained in the speech areas, namely: Broca's, supplementary motor, inferior parietal, and posterior temporal regions.

CONFUSION OF NUMBERS WHILE COUNTING

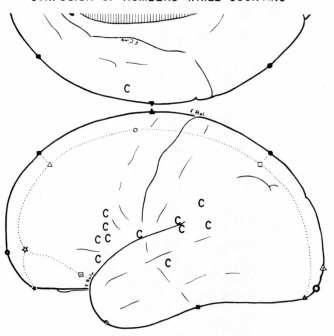

FIG. VIII-7. Confusion of numbers while counting occurred when the electrode was applied to these places. The patient used the word for a number, and not other words, but he counted incorrectly.

Electrical interference involving the right cerebral hemisphere has produced arrest of speech (Fig. VIII-12). Also hesitation, slurring, distortion, and repetition have occurred (Fig. VIII-13). With the exception of two patients, these stimulations are in the Rolandic and supplementary motor areas. Since this review was carried out, one patient has had inability to name with retained ability to speak and misnaming with perseveration during electrical interference involving the right hemisphere. Sometime in the future, it is likely that misnaming without perseveration and confusion of numbers while counting will occur from the right hemisphere.

INABILITY TO NAME WITH RETAINED ABILITY TO SPEAK

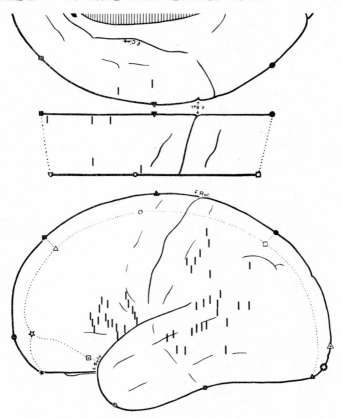

Fɪɢ. VIII-8. The patient could speak, frequently quite well, but he was unable to bring forth the concrete name. One will note that this type of difficulty has occurred from all three speech areas.

B. *Handedness and dominance*

One hundred and fourteen patients (94 and 20 involving the left and right hemispheres, respectively) have had stimulations of Broca's and/or inferior parietal, and/or posterior temporal regions, to determine if speech might be disturbed. These and other patients have had stimulations of the Rolandic and supplementary motor areas, but the number of stimulations producing no effect

127

from these areas is not recorded; therefore, they are excluded from the following analysis. Also, the various other areas of both hemispheres have been stimulated, to determine if speech might be affected. No effect has been noted; however, the location and num-

MISNAMING WITH PERSEVERATION

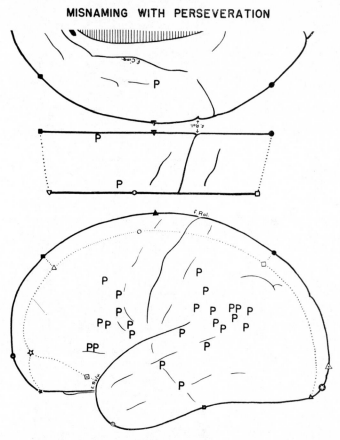

FIG. VIII-9. In misnaming with perseveration, the patient uses a word incorrectly which had been used correctly immediately after or just before the electrode was applied. This type of response has been obtained in anterior, superior, and posterior speech areas.

ber of stimulations is not accurately recorded. It should be mentioned that electrical interference of the left Broca's parietal, and temporal speech areas causes disturbance in speech about fifty per cent of the time.

Ninety-four patients had stimulations of the left Broca's, and/or inferior parietal, and/or posterior temporal regions. Four are excluded from the subsequent calculations for the following reasons: one had electrical arrest which interfered with speech during one operation and stimulations which did not disrupt speech at another

MISNAMING WITHOUT PERSEVERATION
USING SYNONYMS AND UNRELATED WORDS

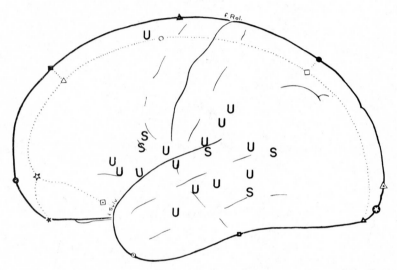

FIG. VIII-10. Sometimes the patient names the picture incorrectly, using a synonym or a completely unrelated word and a word which he has not used in the recent past.

operation; one had interference in speech from stimulation during both operations and had aphasia after one but not the other; two others classed as left-handed had been right-handed before the age of three years.

Fifty-four of sixty-five right-handed patients having aphasia after operation had stimulations affecting speech from one or more of these areas (see Table VIII A). Ten of fifteen right-handed patients having no aphasia after operation had electrical arrests which affected speech. Two of three left-handed patients (or four of five, if those who changed from right- to left-handed are included) had stimulations affecting speech and aphasia after operation. Seven other left-handed patients had no stimulations which caused alterations in speech and no aphasia after operation (all had had birth injuries).

Electrical arrest involving the right hemisphere produced dis-

THE APHASIC TYPES OF RESPONSES

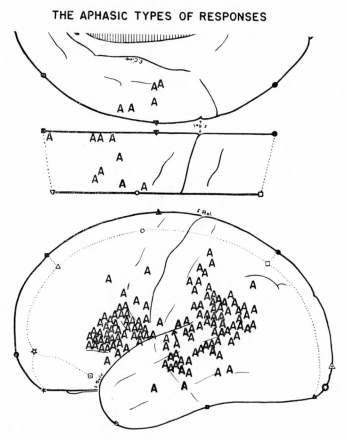

Fig. VIII-11. The dysphasic or aphasic types of responses include distortion and repetition, confusion of numbers while counting, inability to name with retained ability to speak, and misnaming with or without perseveration. Those responses in the central face area are either distortion or repetition of words or syllables, which could be due to a disturbance in motor mechanisms; otherwise, we believe these responses are due to disturbances in speech mechanisms.

turbance in speech in one left-handed patient who had aphasia after operation. Five left-handed patients had stimulations of the right hemisphere which did not affect speech, and they had no aphasia after operation. Of fourteen right-handed patients who had no aphasia after operation on the right hemisphere, one had electrical interference affecting speech.

ARREST OF SPEECH

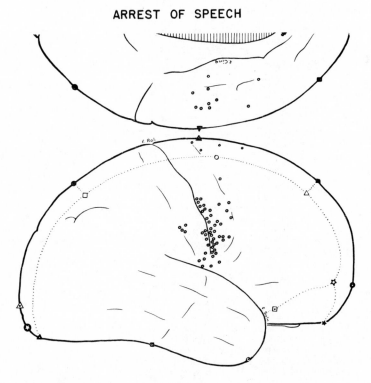

Fig. VIII-12. Arrest of speech has occurred from these points in the right hemisphere within primary and supplementary motor areas.

C. *Discussion*

The positive effect on speech produced by stimulation of the human cerebral cortex is vocalization, which was first noticed by Penfield in 1935. Vocalization is obtained from that part of the precentral and postcentral gyri which yields movements of the lips, jaw, and tongue on stimulation, and also from the supplementary motor area. Vocalization occurs during stimulation of these areas but of no other cortical region in either hemisphere. Brickner (1940), Penfield and Welch (1951), and Erickson and Woolsey (1951) have reported vocalization from the supplementary motor area. Vocalization may also occur from the second sensory-motor area, but as primary and second face areas seem to be in juxtaposition, this is difficult to determine from the old records.

The negative effect on speech caused by electrical arrest is in-

HESITATION, SLURRING, DISTORTION AND REPETITION

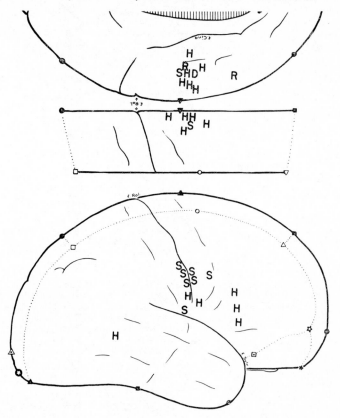

FIG. VIII-13. Hesitation, slurring, distortion, and repetition have occurred from these points in the right hemisphere. The H's in Broca's area and the posterior temporal region occurred in one patient who had some dysarthria after temporal lobectomy, but she had no dysphasia. More recently we have seen dysphasic responses from electrical interference of the right hemisphere, so that we have no doubt that speech representation may be on the right occasionally in both the right- and left-handed.

ability to vocalize or to use words properly. The electric current may cause a complete arrest of speech when applied to those same areas where vocalization is produced. In obtaining arrest of speech from the supplementary motor area, Erickson and Woolsey (1951) have confirmed the results of Penfield and Welch (1951). Because movements of some of the muscles necessary for speech may be obtained from stimulation of these same areas, it is believed that these results are due to an interference with the motor mechanism of speech. Hesitation, slurring, distortion, and repetition of words

TABLE VIII A

Aphasia During Electrical Interference and After Operation

		Broca		Inferior Parietal		Posterior Temporal		Total	
		+[1]	−[2]	+	−	+	−	+	−
Stimulation of left hemisphere	Right-handed Aphasia	46	10	21	13	31	6	54	11
	No aphasia	6	6	3	3	6	1	10	5
	Left-handed Aphasia	2	1	1	0	1	1	2	1
	No aphasia	0	5	0	5	0	6	0	7
Stimulation of right hemisphere	Left-handed Aphasia	0	1	1	0	−	−	1	0
	No aphasia	0	2	0	3	0	4	0	5
	Right-handed No aphasia	1	11	0	5	1	4	1	13
	Aphasia	−	−	−	−	−	−	−	−

[1] + indicates the number of patients who had stimulations affecting speech.
[2] − indicates the number of patients who had stimulations not affecting speech.

occur from these areas; they also could be interpreted as being due to a disturbance in the control of muscles used in speech.

The preceding negative effects, as well as inability to name with retained ability to speak, confusion of numbers while counting, and misnaming with or without perseveration, have occurred during electrical interference of the left Broca's, inferior parietal - posterior temporal, and supplementary motor areas. This is an arbitrary classification of the results noted during application of an electric current while the patient is naming a series of pictures of objects. Obviously, he must have some type of "set" to be able to name. One might expect that if it were just the "set" which influences the naming, stimulation of either frontal region, or other areas, might alter the act, but this has not been found to be so.

The electric current produces effects on speech similar to those produced by seizure discharges. Dysphasia associated with seizures occurs during discharges involving the dominant hemisphere. Difficulty in naming may be a matter of simple forgetfulness, and it has been reported with lesions of various parts of either hemisphere. Perseveration of thoughts and acts is a common finding in the brain-injured. However, it is only during electrical arrest of certain areas of the left hemisphere (on rare occasion, the right hemisphere) that these results have occurred. It is believed that this is an interference with language.

Other parts of the left hemisphere—the frontal and occipital poles, etc.—have been stimulated without affecting speech. However, the number of stimulations is not sufficient to be statistically significant.

In the areas from which effects have been obtained, there is an area-localization and not a point-localization. For example, electrical arrest in the temporal region five centimeters, seven centimeters, and nine centimeters from the tip may interfere with speech; whereas, at other points between them no interference is produced. Also, stimulation of the first, second, and third gyri anterior to the left precentral face area may produce effects upon speech, though stimulation of the same gyri at other points does not. Some of the responses seen in Figure VIII-3 may be responses at a distance, just as Penfield and Boldrey (1937) showed for primary motor responses. We believe that the areas where stimulation will affect speech are those shown in Figure VIII-14, with the exclusion of the motor face area.

Electrical interference in a given area is only effective about fifty per cent of the time. Similarly, stimulation of one point in the motor region may produce a particular movement at one time and no movement on the next occasion,* or else a slightly different one. As we have attempted to show in Chapter V, the left hemi-

---

* This refers to stimulation of one point where a numbered ticket is placed and later removal of that ticket and restimulation—the placement cannot be exact. If exact placement is achieved by a fixed electrode, remarkably constant results are obtained from the motor area and from Broca's area.

---

sphere still subserves speech functions after one part of the speech area has been injured or diseased. We believe that the anatomical substrata for speech are in those areas which remain, where electrical interference produces speech interference. For example, if

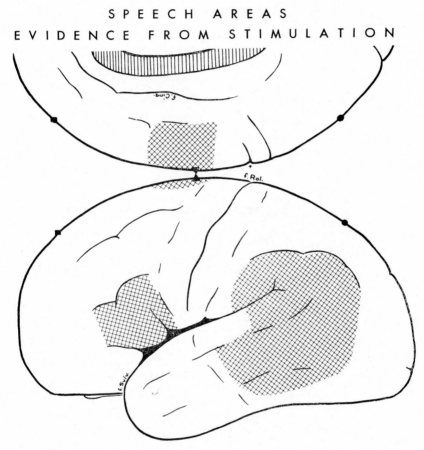

Fig. VIII-14. These are the speech areas of the dominant (usually left) hemisphere. From the results of electrical interference these areas seem to be of equal value.

the left posterior temporal region is destroyed, speech is still subserved by the left hemisphere.

It is not always possible to produce interference in speech by electrical arrest, even though the patient may have a transient aphasia after operation. The surgeon must be aware of this possibility.

So far as can be determined, there is no difference between the effects of the electric current when applied to the dominant Broca's area, supplementary motor area, or parieto-temporal region as regards the various alterations in speech (see Fig. VIII-14). The reason for this lack of difference could be that these three areas are connected by transcortical and subcortical pathways in a single system. An electrical disturbance set up in any part of the system might disrupt the function of the whole system. It had been expected that the functions of the three areas could be shown to be different as a result of different effects on speech produced by electrical interference. With other tests this might happen, of course, but it has not been found with the naming, reading, and writing tests which we have employed.

D. *Summary*

The electric current, when applied to the cortex, produces two effects upon speech: a positive one—stimulation, and a negative one—interference. When the current is applied to the motor areas (Rolandic and supplementary) of either hemisphere, it may stimulate, producing vocalization, or it may interfere, resulting in a disorder of the motor control of speech organs.

When the current is applied to the left Broca's, supplementary motor, or posterior temporo-parietal area (and, on rare occasion, to similar areas of the dominant right hemisphere), perturbation of those processes occurring during speech can be produced. Broca's area consists of the three gyri in front of the lower precentral gyrus. The supplementary motor area lies on the medial aspect of the hemisphere, extending up on the superior surface, just in front of the precentral leg area. The posterior temporo-parietal area occupies the posterior part of the first temporal convolution (exclusive of the auditory area), the posterior parts of the second and third temporal convolutions, the supramarginal gyrus, and the angular gyrus.

The alterations in language produced are: arrest, hesitation, slurring, repetition, and distortion of speech; confusion of numbers while counting; inability to name with retained ability to speak; misnaming with or without evidence of perseveration; difficulty in reading; and difficulty in writing.

SUMMARY

From the standpoint of cerebral dominance, the data from electrical interference support the conclusion, already reached (see Chapter VI), that the left hemisphere is usually dominant for speech regardless of the handedness of the individual, with the exclusion of those who have cerebral injuries early in life.

CHAPTER IX

THE EVIDENCE FROM CORTICAL EXCISION

L. R.

A. *Comparison of excision of atrophic and expanding lesions*

THE practice of using electrical interference and of making planned excisions of functionally active cerebral cortex in the dominant hemisphere, as in the case of C.H. previously described (see Chapter VII), provides evidence of a new type for the study of speech mechanisms and aphasia.

Focal epileptic discharge does not originate in a tumor or scar or an area of gray matter that has been destroyed. It arises in areas of gray matter which are not destroyed but which have been subjected to chronic abnormal influences. The focus may be adjacent to a scar or tumor or to an area of destruction. In any case, its localization is in a zone of gray matter and not just a focal point. Excision, then, is of functional cortex, but this cortex has been functioning abnormally at least to the extent that periodic seizures have occurred.

Surgical removal of tumor growing in the brain may have produced a certain amount of similar evidence, but tumors have a way of involving subcortical structures and also of displacing convolutions to a distance so that it is impossible to identify them. In addition, in most clinics it is the custom to remove tumors with the use of general anesthesia and without using stimulation to identify cortical areas.

The extensiveness of the subcortical involvement and the distortion created by the growth, as well as the frequent occurrence of generalized increase in intracranial pressure, make the use of cases of brain tumor studied at autopsy not the best from the standpoint of localization.

It is true that excision of an atrophic focal area of brain means actual removal of a greater area of cortex than is apparent. Removal of tumor and surrounding brain means often an excision of a smaller amount of cortex than is apparent. The fact that patients with tumor removals have had greater language disturbances than those with excisions of an atrophic lesion may be explained either by the greater subcortical involvement or by the greater involvement of adjacent cortex which is unrecognized, or by some effect of an expanding lesion per se. Similar tumors in similar locations may be associated with different clinical pictures from the standpoint of disturbances in language.

B. *Functional localization*

Judgment of functional localization is based on 1) immediate effect of excision, 2) neighborhood effect of swelling, and 3) late effect of excision.

1. *Immediate effect of excision*

Aphasia occurred immediately after operation on the left hemisphere twenty-two times in 273 operations and did not occur immediately after operation involving the right hemisphere. Thirteen of those having immediate aphasia did not have a tumor and nine had a tumor. Of the former group, four had frontal excisions of the area superior to Broca's area; one had a removal of the Rolandic face area and possibly Broca's area; one had an excision of the area just anterior to Broca's area and the tip of the temporal lobe; five had excisions of the anterior part of the temporal lobe; one had an excision of the posterior inferior temporal region; and the last had frontal and temporal biopsies without cortical removal. It is believed that the reasons for the immediate aphasia are seizures in four, fatigue in three (no difficulty in speech shortly after surgery), vascular occlusion in one (simultaneous aphasia, hemiplegia, and hemianopsia following removal of the anterior temporal region), and unknown in five.

Only three of these thirteen patients had any permanent difficulty. One had the removal of the Rolandic face area and possibly part or all of Broca's area. Two years later he still had definite slowness and mispronunciation in speaking, according to his letter. He has continued to have an occasional seizure. The one with the vascular occlusion had moderate difficulty on examination two months after operation, and still had difficulty eleven months later, according to his letter. He also has had occasional seizures. The third patient had only slight difficulty three weeks after operation. Another patient (removal of the supplementary motor area) died six days after operation. The other nine patients had no permanent aphasia.

Five of the nine patients with tumor who had immediate aphasia had excisions of the frontal lobe superior to Broca's area (possibly involving it in one); two had excisions of the Rolandic face area; one had an excision of the postcentral arm area and the gyrus behind; and the last had the tip of the temporal lobe removed. Seizure with subsequent hemiplegia and aphasia was the cause of the immediate aphasia in two; one had gross brain swelling; and another had fatigue (no difficulty shortly after operation). The latter patient and one with excision of a meningeal fibroblastoma with underlying cortex in the frontal region had no permanent aphasia. The others (all had infiltrating brain tumors) had persistent aphasia and six have died.

2. *Neighborhood effect of swelling*

Most patients classified as having aphasia after operation began to have difficulty in speech one or more days after operation. Frequently, disturbance in speech would be noticed first on the fourth day after operation, would increase almost to global aphasia within the next day or so, would begin to lessen a week later, and would disappear after several weeks. It was assumed, then, that following prolonged exposure to air and ultraviolet rays, as well as numerous electrical stimulations of the brain, physiological or pathophysiological changes (see Prados et al., 1945) had occurred which were different from those seen after ordinary brain trauma. Therefore, we have used the word "neuroparalytic" to describe the edema of these patients. Part of the picture of *neuroparalytic edema* is not paralytic when focal seizures occur in addition to the signs of loss of function, such as aphasia, hemiparesis, etc. This time course was considered most unusual for cerebral edema.

Practically all of the different disorders of language recorded in the literature have been observed in this series of patients. Brief summaries of some individual cases are given below.

In the seventy-two cases in the special study there are not enough cases of excision of one specific area to be compared with those of excision of every other cortical area. The striking fact, however, is that the aphasia, when it occurred, was only transient except in the case of five patients, all of whom have continued to have seizures.

Some twenty odd years ago, and even more recently, it was feared that a postoperative hemorrhage might be present in those individuals who developed aphasia, hemiparesis, and seizures three or more days after operation. A number of the wounds were reopened and no hemorrhage found. No abnormality was noted in many of these, except that the brain appeared "full" or "tense." It was assumed that there was edema. However, frequently the patient had done well for five to eight days.

3. Late effect of excisions

Besides the three patients already mentioned under "Immediate effect of excisions," persistent disturbance in speech occurred in eleven others who had operations on the left hemisphere for lesions other than tumor. Four of them (one frontal, two parieto-temporal and one exploration only) had aphasia after original injury, still had definite difficulty before operation for relief of seizures, had increased aphasia after operation, and had residual difficulty approximately equal to that before surgery. All had continuing seizures.

Another patient (parieto-temporal) had a similar course, except that he had no change in speech immediately after operation and nine months later showed definite improvement, and had had no seizures.

141

Three patients (temporal) in the special study showed only slight difficulty on discharge, and follow-up has not been complete, but they have had seizures. Two others had no difficulty on discharge; yet when one (fronto-parietal) returned to the clinic four years later, his chief complaint was marked difficulty in speech and inability to read and to write; the other (parietal) had his wife write twelve years later stating he had been unable to read or to write since operation. Both have had seizures.

The last of the fourteen patients (CASE C.Y.) had an exploration with transient secondary aphasia. Fourteen years later at the age of twenty-two she had the tip of the temporal lobe removed. Before this operation she had slight difficulty in spelling but otherwise showed no striking difficulty in language, though she appeared mentally retarded. After operation she had a profound aphasia for the second time. She improved before discharge so that she was approximately the same as on admission. The seizures continued, and four years later she had marked difficulty with all tests, except that spontaneous speech was not of the dysphasic type at times other than immediately after a seizure. She had a third operation with removal of the posterior inferior temporal and adjacent anterior occipital region. She showed no appreciable change in language functions after this procedure but continued to have seizures. Four years later she had a fourth operation with excision of the entire occipital lobe. Following this procedure she had transient increased difficulty in naming with perseveration and misuse of words. Whether or not her ability to read and to write will ever return to the point where it is useful remains to be seen. Since the last operation, she has had further seizures and now shows abnormal electrographic discharges in the frontal region. Presumably, this is a case of progressive encephalopathy or encephalitis.

Two patients having operations on the right hemisphere have had permanent speech disturbances. Neither is included in the three patients classed as aphasic. One (left-handed) had a severe accident with evidence of bilateral cerebral damage. When first admitted, he appeared mentally deficient. He had two operations three years apart with excisions of the parieto-temporal region and the precentral face and Broca's areas. No change in speech was noted after either procedure. The other patient (right-handed) had had a birth injury with left hemiparesis and he stuttered. Following a right fronto-parieto-temporal excision, his wound was reopened with removal of a postoperative hemorrhage. He had a decerebrate posture for two weeks and was unconscious for six weeks. He has had marked speech difficulty since recovery but is improving.

C. *Cases*

1. *Excisions in left hemisphere*

CASE W. Oe. A 33-year-old, right-handed man had been struck in the left posterior frontal region by a tool box at the age of 28. He had a small laceration but was not unconscious. Three months later he began to have recurrent seizures. The seizures were characterized by a peculiar sensation in the head, with eyes and head turning to the right, and then inability to speak or to understand what was said to him. At times he would turn around several times to the right. He would then lose consciousness and have a generalized convulsion.

On examination there were no abnormal neurological signs, and repeated electroencephalograms, even with the use of metrazol, showed no abnormality. On testing, the only difficulties were: 1) an occasional mistake when three commands were given (i.e. put your left, third finger on your right eyebrow and your right, second finger on your left ear, and then put your right, fourth finger on your right ear); 2) marked difficulty in repeating the three sentences he reads; and 3) two mistakes in oral calculation (29 plus 36 equals 55, and 16 times 16 equals "132, no, 156").

At operation there was no objective abnormality. The central fissure was outlined by stimulation in the usual manner. Stimulation at point 17 produced something like an attack. He said, "When I have an attack my head turns around like that and I cannot talk." Stimulation at 18 caused him to stop speaking. At 20 he made a number of different sounds but was unable to name. At 18 again, he said, "That is a . . ." but was unable to name. At 22 he was unable to speak. At 25 he said, "This is a comb" (correct), and then said, "This is a . . ." When asked the use of the object shown, just as the electrode was being withdrawn, he said, "to cut," and then named the knife. At 31 the patient said, "This is a trowel," but then said, "This is a hammer," which was correct. Afterwards he repeated, "This is a . . ." several times. After removal of the electrode, he named "a flag" correctly. Points 17, 18, 20, and 31 were in the supplementary motor region, and 22 and 25 in Broca's area. The outline of the excision is indicated by the dashes in the supplementary motor area in Figure IX-1.

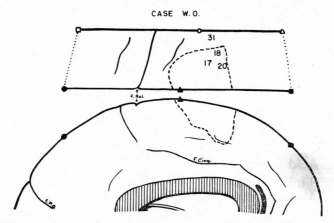

CASE W. O.

FIG. IX-1. Outline of the excision in the supplementary motor area in CASE W. Oe. The numbers in this and subsequent Figures refer to location of points where the electric current was applied—see text for results of these stimulations. This patient had a severe transient secondary dysphasia or aphemia following surgical excision within the broken line.

Following the excision there was some weakness of movements of the right foot. He had no difficulty in speech, naming, or reading. Twenty-four hours later there was the same amount of weakness in the foot as previously. There was no difficulty in spontaneous speech, naming, reading, or writing. Two days later, although he complained of some slowness in thinking and in speaking, there was no obvious defect in spontaneous speech, naming, reading, or writing. The next day, however, there was very marked disturbance in spontaneous speech. He said nothing voluntarily. When coerced, he spoke and had marked difficulty in articulation. In naming he usually mispronounced those pictures that he was able to name; for example, he called bird, "birt," and comb, "homb." He showed evidence of perseveration. Finally, however, he was able to name eight out of ten objects. He had some difficulty in reading letters; for example, g was called "c." He read the word pen as "two" and "dwo" and "too." When asked if it were pencil, he said "Yeh," if it were pen, "Yeh," if it were pencil, "Yeh." He was unable to read a sentence. At that time he was quite fatigued.

On the fifth day after operation the condition was about the same. There was weakness of the entire right side, which was more marked in the foot. Writing with the right hand was unrecognizable. With the left hand he was able to write some words but not others and some letters but not others.

Ten days after operation he showed definite improvement. Spontaneous speech showed evidence of mispronunciation but not of substitution. He named practically all objects. There was slight difficulty in reading. He wrote, "He filped open his big ring notbook and began to read," misspelling flipped and notebook.

On the twentieth day after operation, complete testing showed him to have a very slight disturbance in pronunciation and inflection. He was unable to name a swastika but said that it was German. He made no mistake in oral calculation. In all other tests he did the same as before operation. There was no permanent disturbance in speech from *excision of the supplementary motor area.*

CASE A. Do. A 26-year-old, right-handed man had been in an automobile accident at the age of 19. He spoke immediately after the accident. He had a compound depressed fracture of the left frontal region with laceration of the frontal lobe. Débridement and primary closure were carried out at another hospital. He was unconscious from the fifth to the fourteenth day after operation and then had difficulty in speech for at least three weeks thereafter. His habitual seizures began four months after the accident.

On examination there were no abnormal neurological signs. On testing he had slight difficulty with silent reading, made three mistakes in oral calculation and one in written calculation.

At operation, stimulation of the second gyrus anterior to the precentral just above the fissure of Sylvius (No. 16) caused the patient to hesitate for some time and then to say, "This is a cold." After withdrawal he named comb correctly. The excision included a dense scar with surrounding cortex in the intermediate precentral region above the fissure of Sylvius, as outlined in Figure IX-2. Following a seizure produced by stimulation, he developed slight weakness of the right face, but this was not increased after

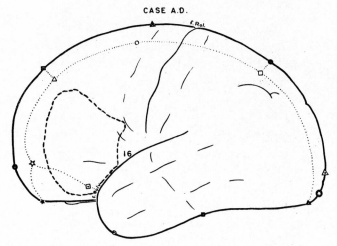

Fɪɢ. IX-2. Outline of the excision in the second and third frontal convolutions in CASE A. Do. He had a severe transient dysgraphia.

the excision. After the excision there was no difficulty in spontaneous speech, naming, reading, or obeying a single written command.

The day after operation there was no facial weakness. He had no difficulty in spontaneous speech, naming, or reading on the first, second, sixth, or ninth day after operation. Complete testing was repeated on the ninth day after operation. At that time he had a little more difficulty with the silent reading, and all other tests were done as well as before surgery except for writing. He wrote, "Well, I thought thing I am going to the ('the' was struck out) tell is about my operation and it is not about all I can tell is about the preparation the had was always the V ('V' struck out) time was when they had me to get ready that is they shaved off all my hair was and a few odd parts of pencil they pr ('pr' struck through) quive me in the fanny.

"My why (both struck through) when they quite me upstair they had me in quite a few places until they had me comfortably and they ('they' struck through) then they were in to the operation room and they asked me all sorts of questions to quite me memory quite quickly and keep it fresh." When given "Around the rugged rock the ragged rascal ran," to write to dictation, he wrote, "Around the rugged rock the rackket rascal ran." No such mistakes were made before operation. Three months later he wrote an excellent letter without mistakes.

Psychological tests were carried out by Dr. Brenda Milner before, and fourteen days, and seven years after operation (see Table IX A).

TABLE IX A

PSYCHOLOGICAL TESTS BEFORE AND 14 DAYS AND 7 YEARS AFTER OPERATION ON A.Do.

	Before	14 days	7 years
VERBAL TESTS	Form I	Form II	Form I
Stanford-Binet Vocabulary (1916)	26/50	19/50	23/50
McGill Verbal Situation (short)*	14/20	9/20	15/20
Wechsler Similarities	8	9	9
McGill 4th Word*			
(verbal analogies)	18/30	15/30	14/30
VISUAL TESTS			
McGill Picture Anomaly—Series 2†	28/34	31/34	30/34
California Test of Mental Maturity			
Elementary and Intermediate			
series (one form)	20/30	21/30	—
Raven Progressive Matrices (shortened)	11/18	13/18	—
Benton Visual Memory	6/7	6/7	—
Wechsler Picture Arrangement	12	11	16
TESTS OF SPATIAL ABILITY			
Wechsler Block Design	15	15	14
Halstead Tactile Formboard (one form)			
1 Mean time for 2 trials	3' 17"	1' 47"	—
2 No. of shapes recalled	4.5	4.5	
3 No. correctly localized	4	4	
Street map showing surroundings of			
patient's house	Good	Excellent	Excellent
MISCELLANEOUS TESTS			
Wechsler Digit Span	7	9	10
Wechsler Digit Symbol	13	9	11
Porteus maze	15.5 yrs.	16 yrs.	18 yrs.
Story recall	10.5		12

All results of Wechsler's tests are given in weighted scores; over 10 is above average performance.

* Hebb (1942b)
† Hebb and Morton (1943)

All performance tests were above the average level and remained at about the same level, except Digit Symbol which dropped sharply as did the patient's writing ability fourteen days after operation. Verbal tests were at average or low average level before operation and all but one deteriorated. Seven years later he had returned to his ability before operation in the McGill Verbal Situation Test; he had improved in Stanford-Binet Vocabulary, but not to his previous ability; no improvement was noted in the McGill 4th Word Test (however, some deterioration is found with increasing age). Story recall, on the other hand, had shown definite improvement from normal (10.5) to superior (12) level.

Partial *excision of the second and third frontal convolutions* was followed by a transient dysgraphia and lowering of scores in verbal intelligence tests.

CASE J. Mo. An 11-year-old, right-handed boy had had seizures since the age of six months. He had some difficulty in speech following major seizures. Neurological examination revealed no abnormalities. Detailed testing was not carried out, but he had no obvious aphasia.

At operation there was slight atrophy of the lower part of the postcentral gyrus and of the gyrus behind it. Stimulation of each of the two gyri anterior to the precentral face area did not interrupt counting. The precentral and postcentral face area and the gyrus posterior to them were removed (Fig. IX-3).

For the first two days after operation there was no obvious difficulty in speech. At forty-eight hours he began to slur and to have difficulty finding his words. The next day his only word was "no," sometimes used incorrectly. He improved, and eighteen days after operation he had no difficulty in spontaneous speech, naming, or reading, but his spelling and writing were rather poor.

As this boy was not tested before operation, his spelling and writing deficits are of questionable significance. It is most interesting, however, that he was not dysarthric immediately after excision of the motor cortex concerned with movements of lips, jaw, and tongue. That this hemisphere was dominant is proved by the transient severe aphasia without hemiplegia.

Excision of the precentral and postcentral face area was followed by transient dysarthria and dysphasia.

CASE W. Pe. A 33-year-old man had had seizures for two and

CASE J. Mo.

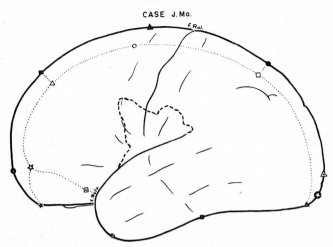

FIG. IX-3. Outline of excision in CASE J. Mo. He had a transient secondary aphasia after operation.

one-half years. He was left-handed, but at the age of six he was taught to write with his right hand. He used a hammer and some other tools with his right hand but ate and did most other things with his left hand. There was a history of stuttering since the age of six years.

Following a shrapnel wound in the left fronto-parietal region at the age of thirty, he had transient aphasia and right hemiparesis. Six months later he began to have recurrent seizures. Psychometric studies carried out at St. Anne's Military Hospital one month prior to operation gave a Wechsler-Bellevue full scale I.Q. of 64; verbal, 72; and performance, 60.

Neurological examination at the time of admission showed increased deep tendon reflexes on the right. There was a skull defect in the left fronto-parietal region. This man was tested for speech disturbances before and after operation by Dr. Preston Robb. He was hesitant in speech before operation.

At operation there was a dense scar in the lower Rolandic region. The gyrus anterior to the precentral face area was yellow and tough. Electrical interference of the gyrus which was anterior to the previously described yellow, tough one (No. 11 in Fig. IX-4) and of the posterior first temporal gyrus produced interference with speech. Excision was carried out of the inferior Rolandic region, the gyrus anterior, and two gyri posterior (Fig. IX-4).

149

CASE W.P.

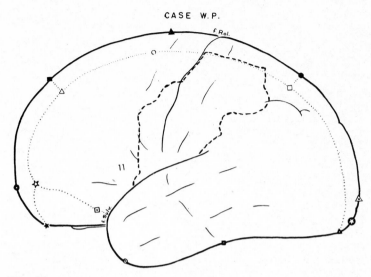

Fig. IX-4. Outline of the excision in CASE W. Pe. He had a transient second-ary dysarthria and dysphasia.

Immediately after operation this patient was able to speak well. Twelve hours later he wanted to ask for water but said "smoke." The next day he became almost totally aphasic and remained so for more than a week. One month after operation, Dr. Robb stated that his spontaneous speech was very good though he still had a slight stutter. He named objects and obeyed commands. His reading and writing were not well done, but Dr. Robb believed that they were performed as well as before the operation.

In this case there was *excision of the supramarginal gyrus, the face area, and Nielsen's Broca's area* (the gyrus anterior to the pre-central face area) without immediate dysarthria and with only transient aphasia.

CASE J. Rl. A 13-year-old girl had had a left frontal lobe abscess evacuated and drained at the age of three years. Two and one-half years later habitual seizures began with initial phenomena of flut-tering of eyelids and turning of head and eyes to the right. Despite medical therapy, her seizures increased in frequency to about three a day. Examination on admission showed evidence of a well-healed fronto-parietal bone flap. There was slight atrophy of the tongue with deviation to the left on protrusion. Dr. Preston Robb found no evidence of aphasia; however, arithmetic and reading were not done as well as the average person of her age would do.

At operation there was a dense scar involving the precentral hand area. The electrographic focus was anterior to the scar. Excision was carried out as outlined in Figure IX-5. Immediately

CASE J.R.

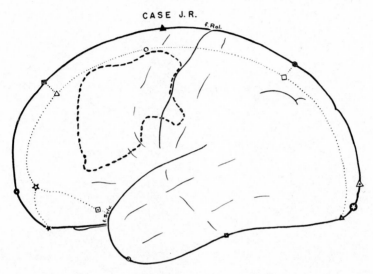

FIG. IX-5. Outline of excision in CASE J. Rl. She had a transient secondary dysphasia without persistent dysgraphia.

following excision she was able to speak but had a flaccid paralysis of the right upper extremity. For several weeks after operation she had marked dysphasia and weakness of the right upper extremity. When seen a year later, she had been free of seizures. Examination showed slight weakness and cortical sensory loss involving the right upper extremity. She continued to write with the right hand and showed no dysphasia or dysgraphia.

Excision of the posterior part of the second frontal convolution was followed by transient dysphasia without persistent dysgraphia.

CASE J. Ma. A 23-year-old, right-handed man had had seizures for six years without preceding injury or disease. His attacks began with numbness of both sides of the tongue, and then he became confused and unable to understand what he heard or saw and could not speak, though he stated that he was aware of something going on around him. Following that, he was unaware of his surroundings and became automatic, looking first at his right thumb and then at his left thumb, or vice versa.

Neurological examination showed no abnormalities. He had no difficulty with any of the speech tests. The electroencephalogram was normal until the onset of a seizure when there were bilateral six-per-second slow and sharp waves in the temporal regions.

The surface of the brain appeared normal at operation. Stimulation of the gyrus posterior to the postcentral face area caused the patient to look suddenly at his left hand, open and close it several times, and then to swallow and to lick his lips. Following that, he was able to talk but then had a spontaneous seizure beginning by looking at the right hand; and a short time later he had a second spontaneous seizure. Numerous stimulations were carried out while the patient was naming, but most of them were associated with electrographic after-discharge. The gyrus from which the seizure had been produced was removed, as outlined in Figure IX-6.

CASE J. Ma.

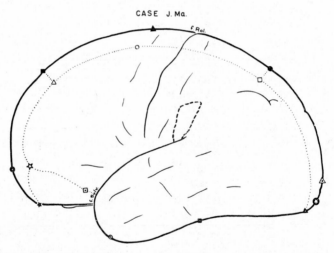

FIG. IX-6. Outline of excision in CASE J. Ma. He had a transient secondary severe auditory verbal imperception.

The day after operation the patient was unusually cooperative and had no difficulty in spontaneous speech, naming, reading, silent reading, repetition, obeying oral or written commands, or writing. On the third day there was slight weakness of the right grip as compared with the left. Although he stated that he was slow, he had no difficulty in spontaneous speech, naming, reading, obeying written commands, silent reading, or oral calculations, but had slight difficulty with the more complicated oral commands. The next day, however, he had moderate difficulty in spontaneous speech and naming, reading, and writing spontaneously. He had marked difficulty in obeying oral commands and in writing to dictation. When asked to write, "The light is poor in this room," he wrote, "The light in the rooms which." He tried again, "The light in the rooms with house." When asked to write, "Those flowers are beautiful," he wrote, "The these flowers the rose kind."

By the next day the patient had practically no spontaneous speech. He was able to write some things that he was not able to say. He by no means understood everything that was said to him; however, he did not believe this. Therefore, dictation was given to his nurse as well as to him and he was able to see the difference. For "The radio is on," he wrote, "a radio even;" for "You do not understand everything," he wrote, "he of understand?" The same type of difficulty was noted in giving him arithmetic to do. He not only mixed up the numbers dictated, but also the arithmetical operation, although he made only two mistakes out of twenty-seven in the actual problems that he finally wrote down. He was able to name only about one tenth of the objects shown, although he could write the names of most of them. He was unable to read aloud, but he had only slight difficulty in obeying written commands.

On the eighth day after operation this patient had two minor seizures of numbness in his lip and tongue. Shortly thereafter he had a period of an hour or more in which he was unable to speak at all or to recognize objects, though he was able to recognize people. Unfortunately, he was not examined in detail during that hour. During the period of time in which he was having so much difficulty in speech, there was no detectable disturbance in sensation or in the visual fields, as judged by simultaneous movements in both visual fields. There was slight weakness of the right hand but no abnormal reflexes.

He showed a rapid improvement, and two weeks after operation the only difficulty found on testing was slight difficulty in oral commands and spontaneous writing. Since discharge from hospital, this patient has continued to have an occasional seizure. It may be pointed out that such small removals are rarely successful in stopping seizures, but the surgeon found no indication for any further excision.

Testing one year after operation showed no difficulty in writing and only questionable difficulty in obeying complicated oral commands. A small *removal of the gyrus anterior to the supramarginal region* resulted in no permanent speech deficit.

CASE E. L. This 39-year-old, right-handed woman had had a cerebral vascular accident at the age of 33. She had convulsions at that time and was unconscious for twelve days, following which she had transient speech disturbance.

Shortly thereafter she began to have seizures. In her minor attacks she was unable to speak and stopped what she was doing; she was aware of her environment and knew that people might be staring at her. Following a series of major seizures she would be in a confused state for several days.

Pneumoencephalography demonstrated a cyst communicating with portion four of the left lateral ventricle. At operation this cyst was found posterior to the postcentral gyrus (Fig. IX-7). The cyst was removed, the ventricle was opened, and the pial banks were preserved over the remaining convolutions (Fig. IX-7). She had definite dysphasia for about two weeks after operation. On the thirty-sixth day after operation she had several major seizures with head and eyes turning to the right and with postictal aphasia.

In summary, it has been stated that following vascular accidents the homologous area of the right hemisphere takes over that particular part of language which has suffered with the lesion on the left, such as the understanding of the written word. CASE E. L. demonstrates that following *removal of a cyst produced by vascular occlusion in the supramarginal region* there was again a transient aphasia. The second transient aphasia seems to indicate that *plasticity* of the brain as a result of vascular disease is not different from that occurring after trauma.

CASE D. Da. A 16-year-old, right-handed boy had an excision of an atrophic lesion in the anterior superior part of the parietal lobe, as outlined in Figure IX-8. Two days after operation he began to have difficulty in speech. The aphasia disappeared by the twenty-second day after operation.

In conclusion, *removal of the left anterior superior parietal*

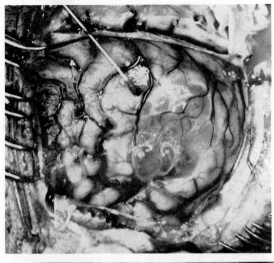

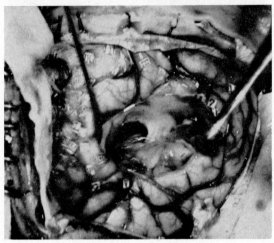

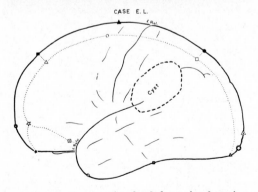

CASE E. L.

FIG. IX-7. Above is shown the cyst in the left parietal region which was produced by vascular occlusion in CASE E. L. In the middle is a picture of the brain following removal of the cyst with opening of the ventricle. Below is the outline of the location of the cyst. She had a secondary transient aphasia after operation.

CASE D. D.

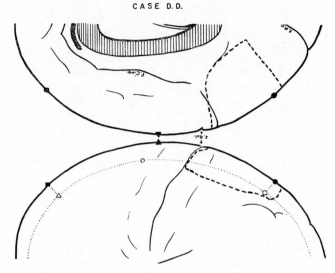

Fig. IX-8. Outline of excision in CASE D. Da. There was a transient secondary aphasia.

region produced no aphasia until the third postoperative day when transient aphasia occurred.

CASE P. A. This 23-year-old, right-handed Canadian Indian was admitted to the Montreal Neurological Institute in January, 1956, complaining of seizures for the preceding eight years. Details of his birth history were unobtainable. He was involved in an automobile accident shortly before or shortly after onset of seizures eight years previously. He was unconscious for thirty minutes and hospitalized for several days. His first language was an Indian dialect and his second was English.

He seemed to have two types of attacks: 1) a sensation of a tickling or cramp in the right instep followed by numbness or tingling in the right leg and body, and 2) a feeling that he was falling towards the left, although he actually did not move, followed by abduction and movement of right arm. In one witnessed attack there was dysphasia postictally. He had one or the other or both minor seizures several times a day, and major convulsions several times a week or several a month.

Neurological examination on admission showed no abnormalities. X-rays of skull and pneumoencephalogram were interpreted by Dr. McRae as showing relative smallness of the left cerebral hemisphere, particularly of the temporal lobe, which he believed had been present since birth or early life. Electroencephalographic studies revealed independent spike discharges from the left parietal parasagittal area and the left posterior temporal region.

The injection of 170 mgm. of sodium amytal into the left carotid artery resulted in transient arrest of counting and right hemiplegia. There was initial confusion, then dysphasia, and finally recovery of the hemiplegia and dysphasia in five minutes. When 170 mgm. of sodium amytal was injected into the right carotid artery, the patient continued to count after injection. There was initially a left hemiplegia and confusion. There was no evidence of dysphasia. From these tests it was concluded that speech representation was in the left hemisphere.

At operation no abnormality was seen on the surface. Stimulation of the postcentral gyrus at the midline produced his first type of attack with sensation in the foot (Fig. IX-9). The superior parietal region was then removed. Independent spiking was found in supramarginal, angular, and posterior first temporal convolutions. This area was then removed slowly with the patient talking continually, and there was no disturbance in speech at the end of the excision. The outline of the removal is seen in Figure IX-9. The tissue removed was tough and abnormal. Microscopically there was focal neuronal degeneration with slight gliosis.

Twenty hours after operation he began to have some dysphasia. This deficit increased so that he had only a few words remaining to him and there was considerable perseveration. He began to improve eleven days later but still had some difficulty in all spheres of language on discharge, twenty days after operation. He has not returned for follow-up, but, according to a letter from a nurse in the Department of National Health and Welfare in New Brunswick, he is doing well, but at times he finds it hard to remember names.

In summary, this man began to have seizures at the age of fifteen, eight years before surgery. He had no dysphasia at the outset. This radical removal was undertaken with trepidation by Dr. Rasmussen; but, as the patient continued to speak well his second and less efficient language—English—most of the parietal lobe

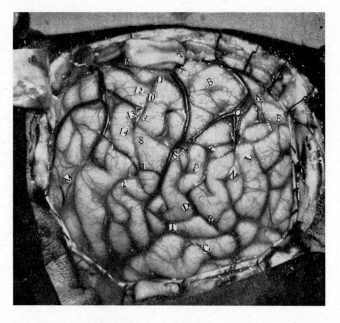

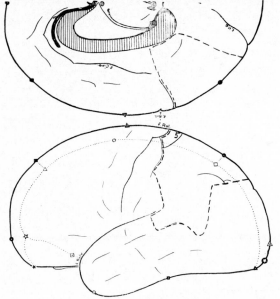

FIG. IX-9. Above is seen the exposed brain, which is grossly normal, in CASE P. A. Points 14, 13, and 12 are on the precentral gyrus; points 2, 1, 8, 3, 10, 11, 4, 7, and 5 are on the postcentral gyrus. The letters show where there were abnormal electrical discharges. Below is seen the outline of the excision. He had a transient severe secondary aphasia.

158

was removed. The microscopic sections showed definite nerve cell damage, but the cause of these changes is not clear.

The fact that the day after operation he developd dysphasia which progressed to an almost global aphasia indicates that the left hemisphere was dominant for speech, thus confirming the results obtained by intracarotid arterial injection of sodium amytal.

Even though there is no gross abnormality, *excision of most of the parietal lobe* may be performed without persistent gross dysphasic disturbances.

CASE P. Rx. This 19-year-old boy had had seizures for two years before admission. At the age of 14 months he suffered a head injury. He may have had some speech disturbance at that time. At the age of 19 he used both his left and right hands and considered himself ambidextrous.

His seizures began with a sensation of numbness all over, and then he believed that men were around him and were saying evil things about him; following this he would lose consciousness.

At operation there was a dural defect with erosion of the inner table of the skull over the left supramarginal and angular gyri (Fig. IX-10). His aura was not reproduced by stimulation. Removal was carried out as outlined in Figure IX-10. He spoke well at the end of this operation. Dysphasia began twenty-four hours after operation and lasted for about a week.

In summary, there was probably a depressed fracture at the age of 14 months, as there was a dural deficiency at the age of 19 years. The bone evidently sprang back, as there was no bony depression at operation. The contact of the brain produced the moth-eaten appearance of the under surface of the skull.

He was so young that language had just begun to develop. His handedness was not established at that age, and afterwards he used both hands. Following excision of supramarginal and angular gyri there was no immediate dysphasia. However, two days after operation he had definite difficulty in language, thus establishing the left hemisphere as dominant for the various components of speech. This deficit cleared in about a week.

Following removal of the *angular gyrus and the posterior part of the supramarginal gyrus* there was only transient aphasia which made its appearance on the day following operation.

CASE L. Jo. A 22-year-old, right-handed man had had seizures

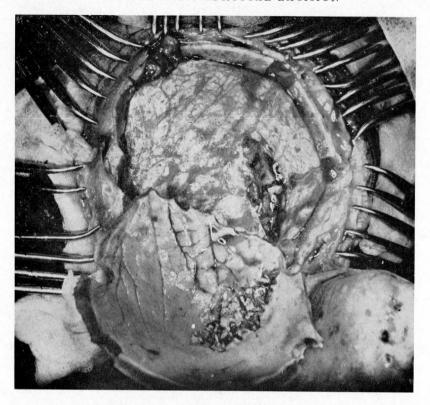

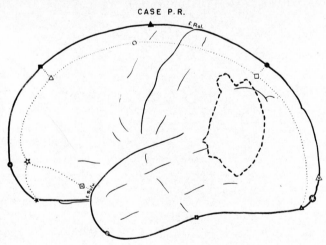

CASE P.R.

FIG. IX-10. Above is the dural defect and area of bony erosion in CASE P. Rx., and below is the outline of the excision. He had transient secondary aphasia after operation.

since the age of five years. Examination on admission showed slight underaction of the right side of face and increase of the right knee jerk as compared with the left. Speech was normal, but special tests were not done.

At operation there were adhesions and an atrophic gyrus in the posterior superior parietal region directly beneath a scar in the scalp. The posterior superior part of the parietal lobe was removed, as outlined in Figure IX-11.

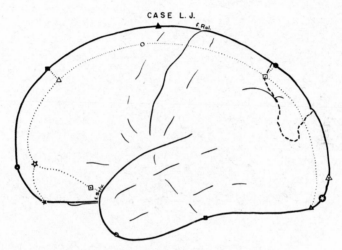

CASE L. J.

F<small>IG</small>. IX-11. Outline of excision in CASE L. Jo. He had a transient secondary aphasia.

There was no difficulty in reading, naming, or speaking with repeated tests until four days after operation. By the fifth day the only words which remained to him were "oui" and "non," sometimes used inaccurately. He began to improve a couple of days later.

Twenty-five days after operation he had no difficulty with any of the tests except slight difficulty in spelling, reading, and spontaneous writing. As these tests were not given before operation, it cannot be stated with certainty that this remaining difficulty was the result of cortical removal.

Excision of posterior superior parietal region was followed by transient dysphasia.

CASE D. Ha. An 18-year-old, right-handed boy had had seizures associated with inability to speak since the age of three and one-half years. Examination at the time of admission in 1932 showed no abnormal neurological signs and no obvious disturbance in speech.

At operation an incision was made into the two gyri anterior to the precentral face area, and a moderate amount of white matter was removed by suction (Fig. IX-12). Disturbance in speech began

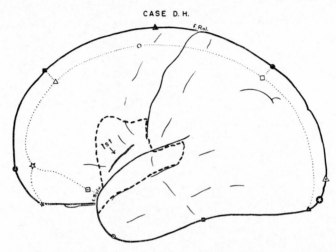

CASE D. H.

Fig. IX-12. The line marked 1st shows the place of cortical incision with removal of an hamartoma subcortically in CASE D. Ha. He had transient secondary aphasia. Ten years later Broca's area, adjacent precentral gyrus, and the first temporal convolution were removed without any speech or other disturbance later.

the second day after operation, and he had a transient severe aphasia and hemiparesis which cleared in a few weeks.

His seizures continued. He returned ten years later at the age of 28 years. At the second operation the lower end of the precentral gyrus and the three gyri anterior to it as well as the anterior half of the first temporal convolution were removed. Following this procedure he had no speech difficulty and no other sign of neuro-paralytic edema.

He died accidentally three years later. At autopsy there was no evidence of tumor. The lack of evidence of growth during the ten years between the two operations, and review of the pathological sections have led us to the conclusion that this was not an astrocytoma (so-called at the time of both operations), but a hamartoma.

This is the only case of *complete removal of Broca's area* in a man whom we might have expected to be aphasic. It would seem that the congenital abnormality had caused displacement of function. That the left hemisphere still functioned during speech is proved by the transient aphasia following the first operation. If Broca's area had been functioning during speech, one might have expected at least some disturbance in speaking immediately after operation, but there was none until the second day.

That there was no aphasia following the second operation does not prove that the right hemisphere had become dominant for speech. The short time required for speech to return to normal after the first operation would indicate that no new area was being trained to be used during speech. Because there was no other evidence of neuroparalytic edema, we would assume that the left hemisphere was still dominant for speech after the second operation.

CASE J. Ch. This 21-year-old, right-handed man was admitted to the Montreal Neurological Institute in August, 1942, complaining of seizures during the preceding six months. Two years previously he had been struck over the left side of the head when involved in a truck accident in Iceland. He was unconscious for thirty minutes, but was back on duty the next day. A year later, during an air raid in England, he was struck in the left temporal region without loss of consciousness. He recalled no difficulty in speech after either accident.

His seizures were sometimes preceded by an aura of epigastric distress, or of dizziness. In minor attacks he had brief loss of consciousness with automatic behavior. He also had major convulsions.

Examination was within normal limits except for a palpable depression in the left parieto-temporal region of the skull.

At operation the dura was found to be lacerated over the posterior Sylvian region (Fig. IX-13). A piece of bone about two cm. in diameter had been driven into the brain about one cm. The area removed included five cm. of the first temporal convolution and the precentral and postcentral gyri, as outlined in Figure IX-13.

Dr. Rasmussen noted in the history: "The patient had normal speech for about 18 hours, and then during the next 12 hours or so developed a practically complete aphasia." By the twenty-first day after operation, dysphasia was apparent only on testing more

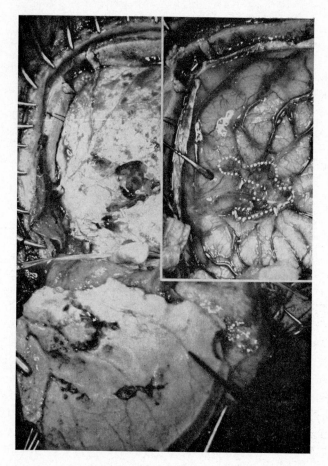

CASE J. C.

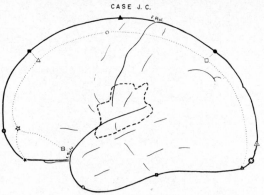

Fig. IX-13. The upper picture shows the dural defect above on the left and the bony erosion below. On the right above is seen the scar in the brain and the outline of the proposed removal. Below is seen the outline of the excision, which was followed by transient secondary dysphasia and dysarthria in CASE J. Ch.

complicated speech functions. Three years later, in answer to a questionnaire, he stated that he had not had a seizure since operation; his letter showed satisfactory use of language.

In summary, either two years or one year before operation, this man had a depressed skull fracture which went unrecognized. He may have had some facial weakness and speech disturbance which also went unrecognized. At any rate, following removal of parts of the precentral and postcentral face area and of the first temporal convolution, there was no immediate difficulty in the understanding of speech or in its execution. On the second day after operation he had a global aphasia. It is permissible to assume that the adjacent areas of cortex were temporarily not functioning normally at that time.

The lower Rolandic region and part of the first temporal convolution were removed with only transient secondary aphasia.

CASE J. Mc. A 14-year-old, right-handed girl had had measles and a generalized convulsion at the age of nine years. Three months later she began to have habitual seizures. The attacks consisted of a sensation in the mid-sternal region, then urinary urgency, salivation, and automatism. Following the attacks she had difficulty in speech and might use unintelligible words.

Neurological examination showed no abnormality. X-rays of the skull showed slight smallness of the left side of the skull with elevation of the left petrous pyramid. The pneumoencephalogram showed slight ventricular dilatation without focal deformity. The electroencephalogram showed two-per-second slow waves and spikes from the left temporal region, transmitted to the right. Testing showed that she had slight difficulty in obeying oral commands, reading aloud, spontaneous writing, and oral calculations. She had moderate difficulty in spelling and in silent reading. Her parents stated that she had had more difficulty than normal in learning to read and to spell.

At operation there was abnormality of the anterior end of the first temporal convolution, in the gray matter adjacent to the insula, and in the uncus and hippocampus. No stimulations were carried out while the patient was naming. The anterior five centimeters of the temporal lobe were amputated (Fig. IX-14). At the end of the operation and during the first twenty-four hours thereafter she had no difficulty in spontaneous speech, naming, reading,

CASE J. Mc.

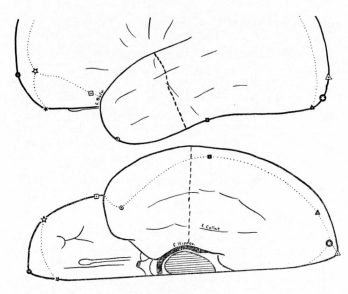

Fig. IX-14. Outline of excision in CASE J. Mc. She had a transient secondary aphasia which was greater than is usually seen after this type of removal.

or obeying written commands. There was no weakness and there were no abnormal reflexes, and the visual fields were full to gross testing.

Thirty-nine hours after operation she was speechless and perseverated on the single sound "owl." How much she understood was difficult to say. She took objects handed to her but did not show their use. She did not obey any written command and was unable to point to any object after reading its name. There was slight weakness of the right side of the face and the right hand. From the third to the eighth day after operation she had a number of minor seizures consisting of movements of the right face, smacking of the lips, turning of the head to the right, and sometimes movements of the right hand.

On the fourth day after operation she said nothing that was intelligible. She was unable to name any object. She pointed to some objects when the name was said to her, and she pointed to all objects after she read the word on a card. She was unable to write with her right hand because of weakness; she wrote her name with her left hand but was not able to write the alphabet. She was able to obey some simple oral commands. When shown pictures of an apple, fish, house, hat, and cow, and asked to indicate those good to eat, she picked out the apple and the fish.

Two weeks after operation she showed some improvement. She was able to say a few words and an occasional sentence, but used many incorrect words. She was able to name only three objects of the entire group, but she usually indicated the correct one when given a choice of names. She was able to repeat some words and sounds, but not others. She read some words and letters aloud and most numbers. She executed half of the written commands correctly. She wrote the names of the objects repeated or shown to her. She was unable to write a sentence spontaneously or to dictation.

Three weeks after operation she showed definite improvement. She had moderate difficulty in spontaneous speech and in naming objects shown to her. She was unable to name any object placed in either hand or to identify sounds by name. There was marked difficulty in executing oral commands and moderate difficulty with written commands and reading aloud. She had only slight difficulty with oral and written calculations.

Twenty-five days after operation she had no abnormal neurological signs. In comparison with the tests before operation, she showed slightly more difficulty in spontaneous speech, naming, repeating, executing oral commands, reading aloud, and writing spontaneously. All other tests were the same as before operation. Two-and-a-half months after surgery a letter showed a number of defects in spelling—about the same as before operation. She had continued to have occasional seizures.

This young girl had always had difficulty in reading and in spelling. Following *temporal lobectomy* she had secondary aphasia. By the time of discharge she had not returned quite to her preoperative ability, probably due to abnormally functioning brain associated with numerous seizures after operation.

CASE H. N. A 19-year-old boy had had seizures since the age of 11. Six months before the onset of the attacks he struck his head in a fall, but was not unconscious. The pattern of his attacks consisted of an auditory aura, then a dream, a tonic, clonic seizure, and post-ictal difficulty in speech, reading, and writing. Neurological examination showed no abnormalities. Pneumoencephalogram showed the left temporal horn to be slightly larger than the right. Repeated electroencephalograms revealed independent abnormal discharges in both temporal lobes. Testing demonstrated no abnormalities except for slowness of speech.

At operation, stimulation of the left first temporal convolution produced both the auditory aura and the dream. The first temporal and Heschl's convolutions were yellow and tough; 9 cm. of the first temporal and Heschl's convolutions were removed (Fig. IX-15). Prior to removal he had some difficulty in speech and in

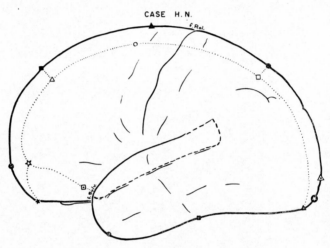

CASE H.N.

Fɪɢ. IX-15. Outline of excision in CASE H. N. There was no immediate difficulty in understanding the spoken word, but there was a delayed transient severe aphasia.

naming, following a seizure. There was no increase in this difficulty after excision. The next morning he had no difficulty in understanding conversational speech, obeying oral commands, naming, reading, or writing, but he had slight difficulty in spontaneous speech. Twenty-four hours after operation he had his first seizure beginning with an auditory aura; he had frequent seizures during the subsequent two weeks.

Four days after operation he was unable to speak or to name, he had marked difficulty writing to dictation, and moderate difficulty obeying oral commands and reading aloud. Ten days after operation his condition was about the same. Complete testing twenty-three days after surgery showed the following changes as compared with the original tests: slight difficulty in spontaneous speech, naming, reading aloud, and writing to dictation, and marked difficulty in oral calculations. Seizures continued periodically after discharge from the hospital.

When tested seven months after operation, he was slow and hesitant in speaking—perhaps, a little more than before operation. He had difficulty reciting the alphabet, getting to "k" and then becoming confused, but finally doing it correctly. He had no, or only questionable, difficulty in all other tests. He was having numerous episodes of momentary lapses of contact with his environment. It is believed that his residual difficulty is related to the frequent minor seizures. *Excision of the entire first temporal convolution* was followed by transient dysphasia.

CASE M. F. A 32-year-old, right-handed man had been in an automobile accident two years previously. He had fractures of the left parietal bone and the base of the skull. He was unconscious or irrational for sixteen days. Habitual seizures began nine months later.

Examination on admission showed no abnormal neurological sign and no obvious difficulty in speech.

Excision was made of the middle part of the three lateral temporal convolutions and the posterior part of the second convolution (Fig. IX-16).

He spoke and named objects without difficulty immediately post-operatively. The next day he began to have difficulty in speech, and this lasted for 30 days. When seen one year later, he had no difficulty in speech.

An *excision of the mid-portion of the temporal lobe* was followed by transient secondary aphasia.

CASE T. M. A 24-year-old, right-handed man was able to do a number of things with his left hand. Several members of his family were left-handed. His younger brother was left-handed and had had definite difficulty in learning to read; he was changed to right-handed and learned to read and to write very well at a special school.

This man had had left mastoiditis and an epidural abscess as a child. He graduated from the U.S. Military Academy at West Point. His seizures began at the age of 22, and he had to retire from the army because of them. The initial phenomenon in an attack

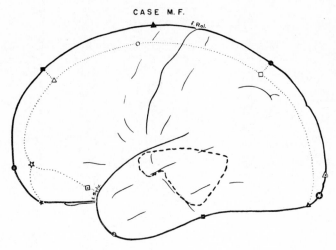

Fɪɢ. IX-16. Outline of excision in CASE M. F. He had a transient secondary aphasia.

was an abdominal aura followed by definite difficulty in speech. Examination on admission showed no abnormal neurological findings. Testing showed slight difficulty in the silent reading test and in spelling.

At operation there were cerebral adhesions and abnormal brain on the under surface of the temporal lobe overlying the petrous pyramid. During electrical interference in the temporal region he had some difficulty in naming. About 7 cm. of the third temporal convolution beginning at 2.5 cm. posterior to the tip were excised, as indicated by the solid line in this region in Figure IX-17. After the excision and before closure of the wound he had no difficulty in spontaneous speech or in reading words and short sentences, but he did have moderate difficulty in naming. For example, a drum was "something you beat on and noise comes out," an apple was "something you eat," and a butterfly was "something that flies." Several hours later he made some mistakes in spontaneous speech and had moderate difficulty in naming and reading aloud. He made one mistake in writing several words to dictation and was unable to execute one of the written commands. There were no abnormal neurological signs. The next day he was practically speechless, though emotional speech, particularly swearing, was present. He was unable to name, read, or obey oral or written commands.

CASE T. M.

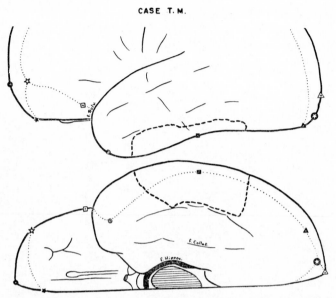

FIG. IX-17. Outline of excision in CASE T. M. He had a transient severe aphasia.

On the fifth day after operation the condition was about the same, with total inability to name, read, obey oral commands, or to select pictures of those objects that are good to eat. At that time he showed slight weakness of the right face and hand but no other abnormal signs.

About two weeks after operation he had improved. He had marked difficulty in spontaneous speech. He was able to spell and to write some things that he could not say and vice versa. He had marked difficulty in naming and in reading, though he was able to read letters and numbers better than words and sentences. He had marked difficulty obeying written commands. He seemed to write a little better than he was able to name or read. He drew a very good plan of the battle of Iwo Jima. At that time he had no abnormal neurological signs.

One month after operation he had slight difficulty in spontaneous speech, naming, obeying written commands, reading aloud and silently, and writing spontaneously and to dictation.

Two months later testing showed no difference from that prior to surgery. Eight months after operation he had one seizure beginning with inability to speak and to name correctly.

In this case there was an *excision of 7 cm. of the third temporal convolution* starting 2.5 cm. from the tip, and only transient aphasia as a result.

CASE E. Ls. This 30-year-old, right-handed man was re-admitted in October, 1956, because of continuation of seizures. He had had minor seizures from the age of 6, and major seizures since the age of 13. He stated that his aura was dizziness, by which he meant a difficulty in seeing clearly. This might be followed by loss of consciousness and falling, or adversion of head and eyes to right, or numbness and weakness of right hand. At times there was postictal aphasia.

In 1942 intracranial exploration was performed at another hospital and no removal carried out. He was free of attacks for one year, and they recurred at a frequency of five to seven per week when first seen by Dr. Penfield in 1949. At operation a calcified mass was removed from the fusiform gyrus. The adjacent part of the fusiform and inferior temporal convolutions also were removed, as seen in Figure IX-18.

He had a smooth postoperative course and only on one or two occasions had slight difficulty in speech.

Again he was free of seizures for one year, and then they recurred at a frequency of about one a week, and with the same pattern.

He was re-operated upon in October, 1956. In the electrocorticogram at operation there was spiking from the remaining part of the inferior temporal convolution as well as from the second temporal gyrus and anterior occipital area. The entire second and third temporal and fusiform convolutions as well as the anterior occipital region to within 3.5 cm. of the occipital pole were removed (Fig. IX-18).

Again he made an uneventful recovery. He had only very slight difficulty in speech, which cleared.

Because of equivocal signs of dysphasia following the three operations, intracarotid arterial injection of 200 mgm. of sodium amytal was carried out on each side. From these tests it seemed quite clear that a profound aphasia occurred after intracarotid

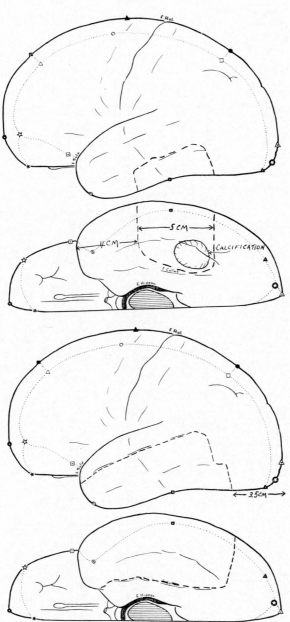

FIG. IX-18. Above is the outline of the cortex and calcification in the inferior temporal region in CASE E. Ls. He had a mild transient secondary aphasia. Below is the outline of the second removal, including the entire second and third temporal and fusiform convolutions. Again he had a very mild transient secondary aphasia. The sodium amytal aphasia test proved that speech remained on the left.

173

arterial injection of sodium amytal in the left carotid, and it did not occur when the right carotid was injected; therefore, it seems that speech was still subserved by the left hemisphere.

In summary, the lesion must have been present before his first seizure, at the age of six years. He had very little dysphasia and no other abnormal neurological signs after any of the three operations, in the last of which there was complete removal of the second and third temporal convolutions, fusiform gyrus, and adjacent anterior occipital area as seen in Figure IX-18. Some might have assumed that the left hemisphere was not functioning for part or all of speech. The results of the intracarotid arterial injection of sodium amytal after the third operation clearly indicate that the left hemisphere remained dominant for speech.

Therefore, in the presence of a lesion dating from early in life, *excision of all of the second and third temporal convolutions* may be performed with only slight transient dysphasia.

CASE C. J. An 18-year-old, left-handed boy had right hemiparesis as a result of birth injury. At the age of 11 years he began to have seizures with an aura of a rotating bright colored light.

On admission he showed smallness of the entire right side of the body below the neck, with spastic hemiparesis, increased deep tendon reflexes, decreased abdominal reflexes, but a flexor plantar response on the right. He had no difficulty in speech.

At operation an extensive removal of the lateral surface of the occipital lobe and adjacent part of the temporal lobe as well as the posterior one-third of the calcarine area was carried out (Fig. IX-19).

He had no difficulty in speech until the third day after operation. He had a transient, rather severe aphasia in all spheres. He still had some difficulty with reading on discharge, but reading returned to normal shortly thereafter.

Despite the birth injury and right hemiparesis, the left hemisphere was dominant for speech. An *extensive removal of the lateral surface of the occipital and temporal lobes* was made with transient secondary aphasia as a result.

2. *Excisions in right hemisphere*

The following three cases are those classed as having aphasia following operations on the right hemisphere.

CASE C. J.

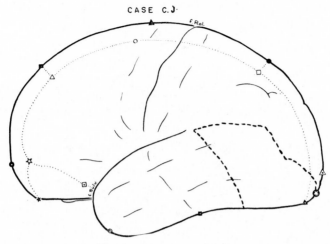

Fig. IX-19. Outline of excision in CASE C. J. He had a right hemiplegia and was left-handed; nonetheless, there was a transient severe secondary aphasia.

CASE A. Ay. A 20-year-old man had had a difficult birth, and seizures during the first two days of life. When he first learned to walk he dragged his left leg. His speech began at the age of 2½ years. He was left-handed, as were his father and others in his family. His habitual attacks began at the age of eleven and were characterized by blurring of vision, nausea, and automatism.

On examination there was a slight left hemiparesis, including the face. X-rays showed smallness of left hemicranium but elevation of the right petrous process. Pneumoencephalogram revealed the ventricles to be moderately dilated, slightly more so in portions 1, 2, and 3 on the left. Electroencephalogram showed abnormal discharges in the right temporal region. His spontaneous speech was fairly rapid, poorly enunciated, and slurred in a careless manner. Testing demonstrated slight difficulty in spelling, repeating test phrases, reading silently, and in oral and written calculation. All other tests were done correctly.

At operation subdural adhesions were noted over the entire exposed right hemisphere, particularly along the fissure of Sylvius. The first temporal convolution and the gyrus anterior to the precentral face area were atrophic and were excised (Fig. IX-20). Several hours after operation there was no evidence of increased weakness, and he spoke, named, and read as well as before. The

CASE A.A.

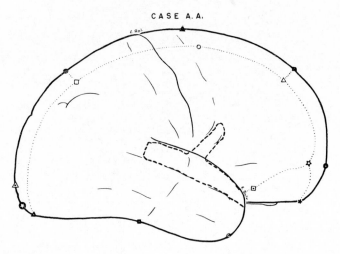

Fig. IX-20. Outline of excision in right hemisphere in CASE A. Ay. He had a transient mild secondary dysphasia associated with generalized increase in intracranial pressure after operation.

next day he was slow in his response and his speech was much more slurred. He read and named a few things and then would not cooperate. Signs of pneumonia appeared on the third day.

On the fourth day he began to have seizures consisting of movements of left face, hand, and occasionally leg, lasting about two minutes and recurring every ten to twenty minutes. They continued for five days and then stopped completely. During that time he did not speak. There was increased weakness on the left, with probably some sensory loss. Deep tendon reflexes were increased bilaterally, more on left; there was an extensor left plantar response and an equivocal right plantar response with bilateral ankle clonus.

On the eighth day he began to improve. Fifteen days after operation, complete examination showed the following changes as compared with the period before surgery: speech was slower; he had moderate difficulty in spontaneous writing, spelling, reading silently, and written calculations; and he had slight difficulty in reading aloud, writing to dictation, and copying.

This patient was examined one year after operation. He had had one series of seizures four months after surgery but none thereafter. His spontaneous speech seemed to be improved slightly as compared with that before operation. Testing revealed no change from before operation except that he had no difficulty with oral calculations.

CASE A. K. A 32-year-old, left-handed man had had a gunshot wound in the right frontal region at the age of 28. The right eye was enucleated and he had complete anosmia. At operation for seizures about 2½ cm. of the tip of the right temporal lobe and a large part of the frontal lobe, which included the entire third frontal convolution, were excised (Fig. IX-21). When the electric

CASE A.K.

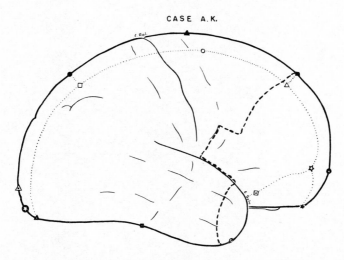

FIG. IX-21. Outline of excision in the right hemisphere in CASE A. K. He had a transient mild difficulty in naming, five days after operation.

current was applied to the second frontal convolution posteriorly, above the area excised, and to the parietal region, some disturbance in speech occurred.

On the fifth day after operation it was noted that he had difficulty in naming objects, though he thought he named them correctly; there were no motor or sensory disturbances. He had no difficulty in naming several days later, according to the record.

CASE W. My. A 15-year-old, right-handed boy had had seizures beginning with inability to speak, write, or understand, though he remained conscious of his environment. At operation there were adhesions over the lower posterior frontal and adjacent temporal regions, and the gyrus anterior to the motor face area was yellowish-gray and atrophic—it was removed (Fig. IX-22).

177

CASE W. M.

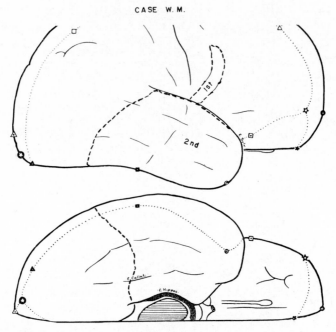

FIG. IX-22. At the first operation the gyrus in front of the precentral face area was removed in CASE W. My. He was reported to have had "nominal aphasia and inability to write," between the fourth and sixth days after operation. This cleared completely. Four years later the temporal lobe was removed. He had no difficulty in speech after surgery, but died three days later as a result of a transfusion reaction.

Between the fourth and sixth days after operation he is reported to have had "nominal aphasia and inability to write." This cleared completely. He continued to have seizures, and four years later the right temporal lobe was excised back to a level 3 cm. posterior to the central fissure if it were extended downwards (Fig. IX-22). He had no speech disturbance but died three days later as a result of kidney damage from a transfusion reaction.

D. *Discussion*

After reviewing the location of the excisions in all these cases without tumor, it seems surprising that dysphasia did not occur more often immediately after operation. This is probably due to the fact that these patients had previous lesions giving rise to seizures. There were only five patients whose immediate dysphasia

178

could not be explained on the basis of fatigue, post-ictal phenomenon, or probable vascular occlusion. The difficulty in language
rapidly cleared in these five individuals. The recovery occurred in
a period of time too short to consider that some other area had
taken over the function of the area excised.

In addition, areas similar in location and extent to those removed
in patients with immediate dysphasia have been removed in other
cases without immediate difficulty in speech. Therefore, we conclude that in this series of patients the brain removed was not in itself
responsible for the immediate aphasia. This argues that the operator had a correct conception of what cortex could be removed in
the individual patient. It must be remembered that the brain removed was abnormal. We do not know what immediate disturbance in speech would have occurred if there had been normal
brain.

From our experience and from the literature it seems clear that
the entire dominant frontal lobe in front of the posterior part of
the third frontal convolution or the anterior two-thirds of the
temporal lobe may be removed in patients with grossly normal
brains without immediate aphasia. It is not clear from the reports
of Bürckhardt (1891) and Mettler (1949) whether excisions in the
temporo-parietal or Broca's area usually will result in immediate
aphasia. These patients were operated upon in the treatment of
psychiatric disorders. Others have had small removals within the
motor areas without immediate aphasia in the treatment of involuntary movements. Other areas of the cerebral cortex have not
been removed in individuals with grossly normal brains—there
has been a tumor, scar, etc., in each.

Our patients were classified as having immediate aphasia only
if it occurred as a result of operation. In other words, if one had
difficulty with language before operation and no change afterwards, that patient was not considered to have immediate aphasia;
there were seven such patients.

Immediate aphasia is known to accompany some cerebral vascular accidents. The cortical area involved is similar in location to
that removed in some of our patients; yet ours did not have immediate difficulty in speech. The explanation of the difference
may be related to the previous damage which gave rise to seizures
in our patients, or to subcortical involvement with vascular dis-

ease, or to unknown factors. We do not know if removal of any specific cortical area would produce constantly immediate aphasia, as the surgeon has avoided those areas which he considered might cause such a deficit.

The type of immediate aphasia was either speechlessness, usually associated with some weakness of the right side of the body, or inability to name objects. The location of the excision did not seem to influence the type of difficulty. The one exception was the patient with frontal and temporal lobe biopsies without further removal. He had what might be called partial auditory imperception. Possibly some damage was done to the first temporal and Heschl's convolutions. These areas, including all of the transverse gyri of Heschl, have been excised in other patients without immediate disturbance in understanding the spoken word. Perhaps the auditory imperception resulted from abnormal functioning of lateral temporal and Heschl's convolutions.

Another surprising fact was the absence of immediate dysarthria in several cases following excision of the precentral and postcentral gyri for face. The gyrus anterior and/or the one posterior to the face area also were removed in these patients. These individuals later became aphasic and then had marked dysarthria in the period of recovery. It seems reasonable to conclude that some other area of the left hemisphere (perhaps the supplementary motor area) was functioning during motor speech, immediately after excision of the central (postcentral and precentral gyri) face area.

CASE D. Ha. (page 161) is the only case of complete removal of Broca's area in a man whom one might have expected to become aphasic. Either the congenital malformation (hamartoma) or the injury to Broca's area at the first operation resulted in other areas taking over its function, or Broca's area is not essential for speech.

It is perhaps easier to understand why immediate aphasia did not occur after excision of the posterior parieto-temporal region in our cases because of the large meningo-cerebral cicatrix or cyst in each. Several patients had marked aphasia with original injury, subsequent improvement, and no definite alteration in speech following a temporo-parietal excision (one of whom was reported by Wechsler in 1937). Three others had a similar history, except that they again had marked aphasia beginning a day or so after excision of the meningo-cerebral cicatrix in the temporo-parietal region.

We have shown that any limited, previously damaged area of the left cerebral hemisphere may be excised with transient aphasia, but without immediate or permanent dysphasia, so long as the remaining brain functions normally. These removals include the anterior two-thirds of the frontal lobe, the entire supplementary motor area, the entire second frontal convolution, the precentral and postcentral face area and the gyrus anterior, the central area for the upper and lower extremities, the superior parietal lobule, the supramarginal and angular gyri, the entire first temporal convolution including Heschl's gyri, the anterior 7 cm. of the temporal lobe including the island of Reil, the posterior inferior temporal region, and the entire occipital lobe—if the outlines of excision are combined, all parts of the left hemisphere are included in the map.

Most of the patients having speech disturbances had transient aphasia lasting no more than several weeks. Because areas similar to those removed in the fourteen patients who had a permanent disturbance in speech have been removed in other patients without producing a permanent defect, and because all patients who have had a persistent disturbance in speech have continued also to show evidence of abnormally functioning brain with seizures, etc., it is concluded that the brain removed is not in itself responsible for the permanent defect. On the other hand, a patient had aphasia after original injury and residual dysphasia before parieto-temporal excision. There was no particular change in speech after operation, but when examined nine months later, during which time he had had no seizures, speech had returned to normal.

Those patients with excision of an atrophic lesion and subsequent neuroparalytic edema may have profound aphasia. In animals, exposure of the cortex to air and ultraviolet rays may cause pathological changes in the area exposed, and even at a distance (Prados et al., 1945). Every attempt has been made to prevent these changes in man; nonetheless, they may occur occasionally. We believe that pathological changes have occurred in the few patients who have had persistent defects in language. If the edema subsides without pathophysiological change, the residual disturbance in language has been little or none in these cases.

In this series of patients the frequency of transient dysphasia was significantly less after excision of the left frontal pole or only exploration of this hemisphere. Following excision of various other parts of the left hemisphere, transient disturbance in language occurred not more frequently after excision of any one area as compared with another.

It should be remembered that these patients were operated upon because they had brain functioning abnormally to the extent that it had been giving rise to seizures. There were at least seven patients who had dysphasia before operation; this number probably would have been higher had all patients been examined in detail from the standpoint of language. The location of the excision in these seven was left frontal in one, temporo-parietal in three, temporo-occipital in one, no excision in one, and involvement of the right hemisphere in the last. The latter is the left-handed patient referred to on page 142 who had no change in speech following two extensive removals in the right frontal, parietal, and temporal areas. The others had increased difficulties in speech after operation, with the exception of one who had no change immediately and nine months later showed improvement.

In monkeys, also, abnormally functioning brain may give rise to a greater deficit than excision of the same area, as demonstrated by Morrell, Roberts, and Jasper (1956). In these experiments alumina gel discs were placed over various cortical areas and chronic epileptogenic lesions were produced. Normal alpha rhythm in the electroencephalogram is blocked by a flashing light—unconditioned stimulus. If a click precedes the unconditioned stimulus, the monkey can be conditioned to the auditory stimulus with the result that the alpha rhythm is blocked by the click. When an epileptogenic lesion is produced in each posterior temporal region, the monkey is no longer able to be conditioned to an auditory stimulus. If a large removal is then carried out, of not only the area beneath the disc but of surrounding cortex as well, the animal may be conditioned again to the auditory stimulus.

In the special study there were not enough cases in any one group (except for the temporal lobe excisions) to allow comparison of the type of transient dysphasia following excision of various particular areas, one with the others. We do know that certain areas may be removed with impunity, provided the remaining brain functions normally.

All of the frontal lobe anterior to one or two gyri in front of the precentral face area has been removed without persistent dysphasia. There has been nothing striking about the transient dysphasia which may occur, except for the greater expressive difficulty.

The entire supplementary motor area has been excised without permanent dysphasia. Patients with this removal had, among other things during the course of their transient difficulties, a "disorder of rapid and complex movements," as described by Ethelburg (1951) for both speech and other movements and by Penfield and Welch (1951) for movements other than speech.

The Rolandic face area and the gyrus anterior (Nielsen's Broca's area) may be removed without permanent aphasia. The transient disturbance includes dysarthria and other difficulties such as those described by Head in his verbal aphasia. The dysarthria may begin not immediately but several days after surgery. This tardiness of onset may be related to the fact that the area was previously damaged.

Excision of the second frontal convolution may be followed by only transient disturbance in writing and other aspects of language. Removal of the precentral and postcentral gyri above the face area may be followed by transient aphasia.

Except for the single complicated case of excision of an hamartoma involving Broca's area, complete removal of the posterior part of the dominant left third frontal convolution has not been carried out in this series of patients. Mettler (1949) claims that bilateral removal of Broca's area does not produce aphasia; the area removed was not identified by stimulation or at autopsy. Jefferson (1950) also states that he has removed Broca's area without aphasia but does not give the means of identification. Whether or not Broca's area is essential for speech in the adult has not been solved conclusively. When defined as Nielsen (1946) does, namely: one gyrus in front of the precentral face area, it can be removed with only very transient aphasia. We believe that probably the entire third frontal convolution can be excised in the adult with only transient aphasia, provided the remainder of that hemisphere is functioning normally.

The anterior 7 cm. of the temporal lobe including the island of Reil may be removed with only transient aphasia. The type of disturbance in language after temporal lobectomy has varied, but usually there has been transient global aphasia. The prolonged deficits seen with tumors and vascular disease have not occurred with excision of atrophic temporal lesions. So far, we have not been able to correlate the earliest sign of aphasia to appear or the last to disappear with the site of the lesion.

The entire first temporal convolution, the supramarginal and angular gyri, and the entire occipital lobe may be removed with only transient dysphasia. There have not been enough cases studied in detail with any of these three excisions to determine the character of the transient disorder in language.

One is, of course, impressed by individual cases, as, for example, the marked difficulty that J. Ma. (page 151) had in the comprehension of spoken speech following excision of part of the supramarginal gyrus. The neighboring cortex probably was functioning abnormally at that time. However, after removal of at least part of this neighboring cortex in H. N. (page 167), we do not find quite the same type of disorder.

The difficulty in writing after excision of parts of the second and third frontal convolutions in A. Do. (page 145) is striking. We would have considered this as almost an isolated defect if we were relying entirely on the simple tests used, but the more comprehensive psychological tests showed profound changes in the realm of language at that time. Citation could be made of the marked difficulty in reading associated with an occipital lobe tumor, or of the marked dysarthric disturbances noted in a man with a tumor of the precentral face area, but we do not have the detailed psychological testing to demonstrate how many other defects might have been present.

So far as our excisions demonstrate, any limited previously damaged area of the dominant left hemisphere may be excised without producing either immediate or permanent aphasia—providing the remaining brain functions normally.

If the patient has an extensive lesion of the left cerebral hemisphere before the age of two years (and perhaps much older), then the entire left hemisphere may be removed without permanent aphasia, but there may be low scores in some verbal intelligence tests. Exactly how much of the dominant left cerebral hemisphere may be excised in the normal adult without a permanent disturbance in speech is unknown. Zollinger's (1935) case of left hemispherectomy for tumor in an adult demonstrates that some speech may return. However, the patient did not live long enough to determine whether language would have been useful. Also, Hillier (1954) has removed the left hemisphere for tumor in a 13-year-old boy and some language function returned. Our case, C. Y. (page 142), has some useful speech, but reading, writing, and arithmetic are extremely poor after complete removal of the left temporal and occipital lobes, and abnormally functioning brain remains.

The fact that the patient had aphasia with initial injury, and again has aphasia after operation for excision of the scar, indicates that the left hemisphere still functions during speech in these cases. Numerous authors have assumed that the homologous area of the opposite hemisphere took over the function of the damaged one. The literature has been searched to find a satisfactory case of aphasia from a lesion of the left half, recovery, and then a second attack of aphasia from disease of the right half—none has been found. Cases such as that of Bramwell (1898) are evidence to us of pseudobulbar palsy with motor weakness of the muscles necessary for articulation; language is intact. If bilateral removal of Broca's area, as Mettler (1949) claims, does not produce permanent aphasia, then some other area than the opposite Broca's must be functioning during motor speech. Bilateral destruction of the posterior Sylvian area causes difficulty or complete loss of hearing; however, there is no evidence that the second lesion on the right produces disturbance in language.

Our evidence shows that difficulty in understanding speech, for example, is present again after cortical excision in the parieto-temporal region, as it was after injury. We have no clear evidence that only one aspect of speech is taken over by the other hemisphere. Nor is there such evidence in the literature.

Lesions in particular localities may result in specific clinical syndromes. Lesions in the region of the precentral face area and of Broca's area may cause dysphasic disorders which are predominantly expressive in type. This does not mean that a center for eupraxia, and another center for movements of the lips, etc., have been destroyed. There is no specific site where what Nielsen (1946) calls the motor engrams of speech are stored. A large part of the cortex and sub-cortex appears to be active during the production of a proposition. The transmission of impulses from the precentral gyrus to all of the complex musculature necessary for speech is certainly occurring; and there is activity in Broca's area or another speech area. There is, however, no localized area for articulate language in Broca's convolution. Broca's convolution is only part of the whole.

Generally, we believe that lesions near the junction of the dominant parietal and occipital lobes may produce dysphasic disorders, with the most pronounced difficulty in the visual sphere. But there is no localized center in the angular gyrus for the recognition of letters, numbers, or words. One of the chief things that has retarded progress is the acceptance of such a concept as that which states that perception is divided into: first, conscious perception of sensory impressions, and second, linkage of content of perception with other images—a process which can be interrupted at one or the other level by a lesion. We have only an imperfect idea of the exact mechanism of perception, and we do not know that it occurs in these two stages. For example, von Senden (1932) demonstrated the prolonged period of time required for the appreciation of visual cues in older children who had had congenital cataracts removed. These children were unable to use the visual data, even though the visual apparatus was intact, until they had had a number of weeks of exposure to visual cues.

Theory is indispensable, but terms such as those of agnosia, particularly when subdivided into visual verbal, visual literal, etc., do nothing but confuse us. There is not a single case in the literature of visual verbal agnosia without other defects, together with the ability to recognize some word at some time if the examination is detailed enough. We must record what the patient sees and does under this and that circumstance, and not use such terms as visual verbal agnosia and auditory agnosia unless these things actually exist, which, as far as we are concerned, has never been proved. From the standpoint of terminology, we prefer Jackson's "partial imperception."

We shall not describe various syndromes which certainly do occur clinically—as Gerstmann's syndrome, and so forth. It should be pointed out, however, that cortical excisions of areas in which lesions may produce such a syndrome have not been followed by permanent defects.

Lesions in similar locations may be accompanied by different symptoms and signs, depending upon the nature of the lesion. The acuteness of onset, the degree of destruction of the particular area, the effect on the vascular supply of the area involved and of other areas—all may influence the resultant symptoms and signs. Riese (1949) has written an excellent article on this subject.

Granted that the nature of the lesion is the same, and the lesion is in the same location in two individuals; the type of disturbance in language may be different. This difference, we believe, may be due to the variation in the premorbid abilities of the two individuals—their spelling, arithmetic, reading, etc., proficiencies. Different types of dyslexias may occur, depending upon what system was used to teach the child to read.

In an individual who has learned two or more languages, if one language suffers with a cerebral lesion, all languages suffer. As Minkowski (1928) and others have pointed out, it is not necessarily the language which was first or best learned that returns first. Numerous psychological factors contribute to determining which language is most disturbed and which returns first, etc. Different languages do not have different anatomical substrata but the same ones.

What role does the supplementary motor area play in speech? Seizures, electrical arrest, and lesions of the left supplementary motor area may produce disturbances in language. When the nondominant supplementary motor area is involved, temporary dysarthria may result. When it is in the dominant hemisphere, dysphasia as well as dysarthria may occur. The entire supplementary motor area may be excised in the dominant hemisphere with no more than temporary dysphasia. Only as a result of knowing the effects of electrical interference was it appreciated that the supplementary motor area might have something to do with speech. Cases were then found, in the literature and in our own files, with dysphasia accompanying lesions in this area (Roberts, 1952).

The supplementary motor area is supplied by the anterior cerebral artery. As is well known, the most important speech areas are supplied by the middle cerebral artery. Parts of the areas supplied by both the anterior and posterior cerebral arteries may be partially "trained" regarding speech. This may vary in different individuals, as witnessed by the presence or absence of dysphasia with lesions in the areas supplied by the anterior and posterior cerebral arteries. When, however, the area supplied by the middle cerebral artery in the dominant hemisphere is destroyed, these areas then are used in speech.

Jackson's dictum that a lesion produces negative effects, and the action of the remaining brain produces the positive ones, needs to be modified slightly. Part of the remaining brain may be abnormal, and this discharging abnormal brain may give rise to certain effects. Hebb and Penfield (1940) stated that some of the signs of frontal lobe damage may be due not to the loss of the tissue itself, but to disordered function in the remaining tissue. Penfield and Humphreys (1940) stated that chronic progressive degeneration may continue in an area of local cortical atrophy over a period of years. Dysphasia may be caused not by the lesion, but by the discharging abnormal brain.

We believe that the most important area for speech is the posterior temporo-parietal region (Fig. IX-23), including the posterior parts of the first, second, and third temporal convolutions behind the vein of Labbé, the supramarginal gyrus, and the angular gyrus. The next important area for speech is that of Broca, including the three gyri anterior to the precentral face area. The supplementary motor area on the medial, and a little on the superior aspect of the hemisphere in front of the precentral foot area is dispensable; nonetheless, lesions here can produce prolonged dysphasia, and it probably is very important if the other areas for speech are destroyed.

If one of the speech areas is destroyed, then adjacent areas of cortex and the other speech areas function during speech.

1. *The mechanism of speech*

The child learns to speak by numerous attempts at imitation of sounds heard and observation of the effects of his vocalizations on his listeners. A deaf child may learn to speak by imitation of lip movements, and a blind one, without the use of vision. However, in the blind, illiterate, and deaf, language is not as fully developed as normally.

We do not believe the theory that changing the handedness of

SPEECH AREAS
EVIDENCE FROM EXCISION

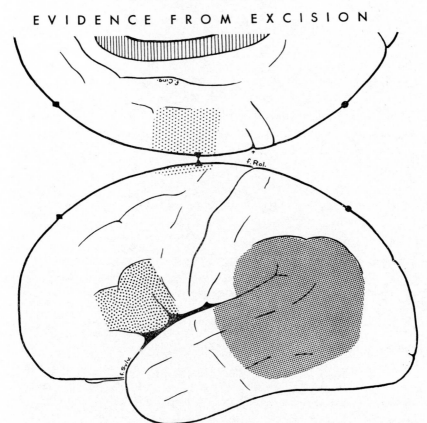

FIG. IX-23. The three speech areas, we believe, are of different values. The posterior, or parieto-temporal, area is the most important. The anterior, or Broca's, area is the next most important but is dispensable in some patients, at least. The superior, or supplementary motor, area is dispensable but probably is very important after damage to one of the other speech areas.

an individual will change the hemisphere dominant for speech. Nonetheless, a blanket rule that because this is a "right-handed world" all should be right-handed is untenable, due to numerous psychological factors—also, what would happen to baseball with the loss of left-handed pitchers and batters! Instead, we advocate greater use of both hands.

We should like to propose the following:

Comprehension of speech occurs after receiving auditory impulses in both hemispheres and in the higher brain stem, and during the interaction of impulses between the higher brain stem and the left temporo-parieto-occipital region. Reading occurs after receiving visual impulses in both hemispheres and in the higher brain stem, and during the interaction of impulses between the higher brain stem and the left temporo-parieto-occipital region.

Impulses produced after interaction between the higher brain stem and the left hemisphere may be transferred to the motor cortex of either hemisphere, and then to the final common pathway to the muscles used in speaking; and motor speech accompanies these transactions. Interaction may occur between Broca's area and the higher brain stem before transfer of impulses to either motor cortex. If Broca's area is destroyed, then interaction may be between some other part of the left hemisphere (e.g. the supplementary motor area) and the higher brain stem before transfer of impulses to either motor cortex.

If the auditory area of one hemisphere is destroyed then that of the other is used alone. Transient dysphasia would result only if the lesion were on the left half, and the cells or pathways connected with the higher brain stem and used during the comprehension of speech were affected. Persistent dysphasia would occur if the latter were functioning abnormally or if the lesion were very extensive. Along with speech therapy for persistent dysphasia, attempts should be made to control or to remove any abnormally functioning brain. In some cases excision of epileptogenic discharging areas will make possible restoration of speech function. The right hemisphere could function for the comprehension and execution of speech only after training.

E. *Conclusions*

1. There are not enough cases in the special study group to allow comparison of types of dysphasia occurring after excision of various specific cortical areas. Nonetheless, it is believed on the basis of individual cases that particular deficits in language may be shown to follow specific cortical removals.

2. Limited excisions of any previously damaged part of the left hemisphere may be followed by only transient dysphasia, provided the remaining brain functions normally.

3. The following areas, as defined in the text, are listed in order

of their importance for speech: the posterior temporo-parietal, Broca's, and the supplementary motor areas.

4. Persistent dysphasia may occur during abnormal function or with extensive destruction of the left hemisphere. Attempts should be made to control or to excise any abnormally functioning brain to allow the patient the best chance for the recovery of language.

5. It is proposed that comprehension of speech occurs after impulses have been received in the higher brain stem and both cortical auditory areas, and during interaction between the higher brain stem and the left hemisphere. Following interaction between the higher brain stem and the left hemisphere, impulses pass to both cortical motor areas and thence to the final common pathway to those muscles used in speech—spontaneous speech occurs during these transactions.

CHAPTER X

CONCLUDING DISCUSSION

W. P.

A. *Retrospect*

In the early half of the 19th century, man believed that the brain was an organ that functioned as a whole, and that all its parts were equipotential. Gall challenged this conception, but the fact that he created an absurd pseudoscience called *phrenology* discredited his anatomical studies. Members of the medical profession looked on phrenology with even greater suspicion when Gall made it both fashionable and lucrative!

In 1861 a French surgeon, Paul Broca, precipitated a widespread discussion of this matter by his description of two patients who had lost speech as the result of lesions in the posterior part of the third left frontal convolution. Nine years later Fritsch and Hitzig (1870) demonstrated by electrical stimulation the existence of a motor area in the cerebral cortex of dogs.

Thus, it appeared that speech and movement had some sort of localization in the brain. Consequently, the physiologists and the anatomists, convinced that there might be many demonstrable and separable mechanisms within the brain, joined the clinicians. The feverish activity which followed has borne good fruit. The young David Ferrier soon hurried to the Royal Society with the excited claim that a scientific phrenology was now to be expected.

But the localization of *speech mechanisms* continued to be the exclusive concern of clinicians. Of course, it could hardly have been otherwise, since man alone, of all God's creatures, possesses this strange faculty. Animals communicate with each other using some sort of meagre language, but only man speaks and writes and reads a language of words. The organization of his brain endows him with the capacity to create and to learn a language. Wherever men have been discovered—in the Americas, Australia, the distant Islands of the Pacific—they have learned to live together and to talk with each other, using a language of their own making.

Russell Brain (1955) summed up a discussion of the origin and nature of language as follows: "Speech is a mode of communication in which symbols are used to convey ideas, to arouse feelings, or to excite actions. In spoken speech these symbols are sounds, in written speech they are visual patterns. Tactile impressions play the part of visual symbols in the blind, and gestures replace spoken language in the deaf and dumb."

Thus, man has devised various means of communication, conveying *ideas* by means of *symbols*. Words are symbols of ideas, whether they are spoken or written or used in unuttered formulations in the mind. Associated with the use of words as symbols, a remarkable lateralization and localization of function has appeared in the human brain. From the point of view of comparative physiology this is a startling event, but no more so than the appearance of language.

The brain of man is not so very different from that of dog or monkey in outward form, but there is within it an altered organization that makes speech possible. It is this structural endowment which forms the subject of our monograph. Thanks to this endowment, man can communicate his discoveries to others and record them in an ever growing body of human knowledge.

In the forty years that followed Broca's discovery, clinicians were coining new words, and at the turn of the 20th century there was a terminology of speech disturbance: *aphasia*, agraphia, alexia, anarthria, aphemia, word-blindness, word-deafness, motor aphasia, sensory aphasia, global aphasia.

General agreement had gradually emerged that the defects in speech described by these terms, with the exception of anarthria,*

* Anarthria may be defined as a difficulty in articulation of words. It is a motor

193

were produced by lesions within one hemisphere—the dominant hemisphere. It was agreed that the left hemisphere was dominant for speech, and that similar lesions in the non-dominant hemisphere did not result in such disturbances. Furthermore, lesions in the central nervous system from the midbrain on down (Fig. II-1) did not produce aphasia.

In the publication of Wernicke (1874) ten cases of aphasia were reported. In two of them (cases 2 and 9) autopsy showed that a vascular lesion had involved the first temporal convolution together with its junction ("anastomose") with the second temporal convolution. "Both patients," he wrote, "suffered from sensory aphasia." It should be added that in each of these two cases there was destructive involvement of the brain beneath the temporal cortex as well—a fact which he did not discuss. Wernicke postulated that there must be, in connection with the auditory area in the first temporal convolution, a word store or *word treasury* ("Wortschatz") which was drawn upon during normal speech. He suggested also that the sound picture ("Klangbild") could be destroyed by a discrete lesion placed more posteriorly.

Wernicke thus described what came to be called *sensory aphasia,* and he localized the causative lesion in the first and second temporal convolutions. But he saw no difficulty in subscribing to another form of aphasia as well—the so-called *motor aphasia*— due to lesions of the posterior part of the frontal lobe, as previously described by Broca.

He drew a number of diagrams (Fig. IV-2) which illustrated his conviction that it was the connections between different speech areas of the cortex that were important, and it was the transcortical connections that he was visualizing. Conduction aphasia, he believed, could be produced by lesions of the connections.

He pointed out, in regard to the other cases, that patient number 1 suffered from almost pure *agraphia* (difficulty in writing). Patient number 3 had largely recovered from difficulty in writing but continued to have a severe degree of *alexia* (difficulty in reading). The location of the lesion in these two patients was not known, as

---

phenomenon and may be produced by a lesion in the motor face-area situated in the cortex of either hemisphere. Anarthria and *dysarthria* are used interchangeably to describe the difficulty in using the mouth and tongue and throat for the purposes of speaking.

both were living at the time of the report. However, he theorized that with greater improvement these patients would become examples of pure alexia and pure agraphia. They would then, he thought, follow the normal evolution of "sensory" and of "conduction aphasia."

This was a good example of the hopeful effort which clinicians have made to recognize pure forms or subdivisions of aphasia, which really do not exist, and exclusively functioning centers of control, which also do not exist.

Thus, Wernicke's name came to be applied to the first temporal convolution (Fig. X-1), as Broca's had been to the third frontal.

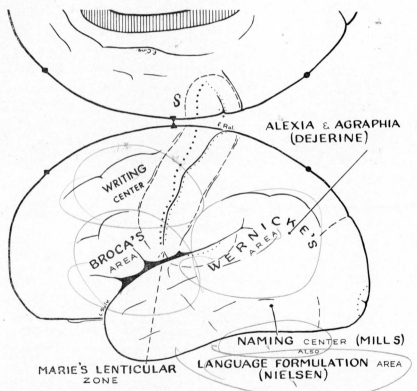

Fig. X-1. Summarizing illustration of the localizations made by various clinicians in the literature of aphasia. S indicates the superior cortical speech area.

But, certainly as far as the evidence from his cases goes, Wernicke's zone should include the posterior part of the second temporal convolution as well, and thus both the angular and the supramarginal gyri, together with possible structures deep to that (Fig. X-2).

Marie (1926) reconsidered the previous work of French clinicians and objected, with some justification, that the attempt to subdivide the aphasic defect had gone too far, that all aphasics had

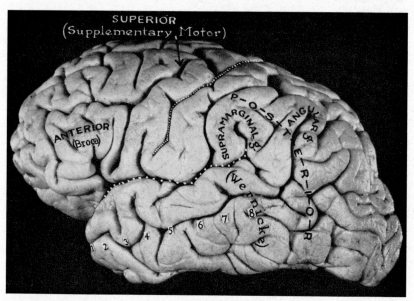

FIG. X-2. On the surface of a normal human brain the areas of the dominant hemisphere devoted to speech are indicated—areas in which local injury or electrical interference produces aphasia. Comparison of this photograph with the photographs in Figures X-5 and III-1 illustrates how varied the fissuring of the adult brain is found to be. Supramarginal gyrus at the end of the lateral fissure (of Sylvius) and the angular gyrus at the end of the superior temporal sulcus are marked M and A, respectively in Figure X-5, and the extensions of these deep fissures are seen in cross-section in Figures X-11 and X-12. A line of small white dots marks the central fissure of Rolando; the larger dots, the fissure of Sylvius. The numbered tickets mark the centimeters from the tip of the temporal lobe backward.

some defect in comprehension—a point of view put forward by Head (1926) in the same year. Marie denied that Broca's area of cortex played any role whatever in aphasia.* He pointed out that a lesion of the lenticular zone (Fig. X-1, also Fig. X-6) produced *anarthria* on either side, and that Wernicke's aphasia was the only true aphasia. It might appear, he said, with or without anarthria,

---

* "La troisième circonvolution frontale gauche ne joue aucun rôle spécial dans la fonction du langage."

depending on whether there was involvement of the lenticular zone as well.

This point of view was not generally accepted by other members of the Société de Neurologie de Paris, and they organized an important series of discussions of *aphasia* in which Dejerine and others defended Broca's belief that a lesion of the posterior end of the third frontal convolution would produce aphasia. Madame Dejerine (1908) supported her husband by pointing out to Marie the importance of the fibers of connection from the posterior end of the third frontal convolution, which would be interrupted by a lesion in the lenticular zone (L, Fig. X-6). These fibers of connection were, she said, independent of the motor fibers in the internal capsule.

The posterior temporal region was subsequently called a *"Naming Center"* by Charles K. Mills, and approximately the same location was entitled the *"Language Formulation Area"* by Johannes Nielsen (area 37 of Brodmann, Fig. II-5).

Stimulation studies within the longitudinal fissure led us to conclude that there was a third area devoted to speech in the dominant hemisphere (Penfield, 1950). It was located on the cortex within the longitudinal fissure (S in Fig. X-1), between the motor cortex for foot movement and the supplementary motor area (Fig. II-10). This may be called the *superior speech area* (supplementary motor).

The summary drawing (Fig. X-1) should serve to recall the observations of many thoughtful clinicians who saw patients with differing symptoms and differing lesions within the dominant hemisphere. These lesions were not on the surface alone. They extended inward in various directions. The patterns of speech disturbance reported by them and discussed in Chapter IV constitute contributions of lasting value.

Many neurologists whose names do not appear in that summary drawing have made contributions of no less importance: Hughlings Jackson, Henry Head, Arnold Pick, Theodore Weisenburg, M. Minkowski, Russell Brain, T. Alajouanine, MacDonald Critchley, and others whose work is discussed in Chapter IV.

Our further discussion will be in relation to the three discrete areas of the cerebral cortex devoted to speech elaboration. These areas are labelled roughly on the surface of a normal brain in Figure X-2 as Posterior, Anterior, and Superior.

B. *Definitions*

Before proceeding it might be well to stop for brief definitions.

Aphasia (or dysphasia) may be defined as a difficulty in the ideational elaboration of speech as distinguished from defective verbal articulation. Aphasia is characterized by the following defects in varying proportions: Ideational defect in speaking, reading, writing, naming, and defective comprehension of speech. Aphasia is usually associated with misuse of words, circuitous substitution of words, *perseveration* in the use of words. (Perseveration is the tendency to use a word improperly which has just before been used properly.)

Dysarthria (anarthria) may be defined as a difficulty in the articulation of words. This may include the motor employment of muscles of respiration and vocalization as well as lips, tongue, and throat.

Speech dominance. The dominant hemisphere or major hemisphere for speech is that hemisphere in which disease or damage may produce aphasia.

C. *Cerebral cortex*

The human cerebral hemispheres are never twice the same in form and in the patterning of convolutions and fissures. Compare the left hemisphere in Figures X-2, X-5, and III-1. At the time of birth the motor and sensory areas shown in Figure II-2 are beginning to take on their function as transmitting stations. At that time the speech areas are blank slates on which nothing has yet been written. In the overwhelming majority, the three cortical speech areas indicated in Figure X-4 will be developed in the left hemisphere (and rarely in the right). But a small lesion in infancy may produce some displacement of the expected location of these areas within the left hemisphere. A larger lesion in the posterior speech area may cause the whole speech apparatus to be developed in the right hemisphere where the cortical areas take up homologous positions.*

* It was pointed out in Chapter VI that a lesion restricted to speech cortex does

We may now summarize our own observations that apply to speech. The nature of our material has been described and discussed in detail in previous chapters. In the cerebral cortex of the human adult there are areas devoted to the control of speech musculature, and there are other areas that are devoted to the ideational processes of speech. Thus, they may be divided into two categories and discussed separately.

1. *Motor mechanisms of speech*

Our knowledge of these areas is derived largely from electrical stimulation of the cortex of conscious men and women.

Vocalization was produced first in the right hemisphere, and later many times in either hemisphere, at a point on the precentral Rolandic gyrus between the responses of hand movement and throat movement (Penfield, 1938). See Figure II-7. Sometimes, when greater detail of response was worked out by repeated stimulation, vocalization was found to be the response of a small area between upper face movement and lip movement (Fig. X-3).

Subsequently it was shown that vocalization could also be produced in the supplementary motor area of either side (Penfield and Rasmussen, 1950). That means that there are four cortical areas in which a gentle electrical current causes a patient, who is lying fully conscious on the operating table, to utter a long-drawn vowel sound which he is quite helpless to stop until he runs out of breath. Then, after he has taken a breath, he continues helplessly as before. Other animals lack this inborn vocalization transmitting mechanism in the motor cortex.*

Voice control. Curious at it may seem, this is the most striking difference between the cortical motor responses of man and other mammals, and it seems likely that it bears some relationship to

---

not cause change of hand dominance, nor does a lesion in the hand area influence the position of speech areas. A large lesion in infancy and early childhood may produce left handedness and may displace speech function to the right hemisphere, but it does so only because both the motor hand area and the cortical speech areas were involved.

* Leyton and Sherrington (1917) observed that they could not produce vocalization in anthropoids by faradic stimulation. Friedman (1934), on the other hand, reported that he had produced a bark by stimulation of the motor gyrus of the dog—an observation that calls for verification. Wilbur Smith (1941) produced some form of vocalization by stimulation of the cingulate gyrus of monkeys,

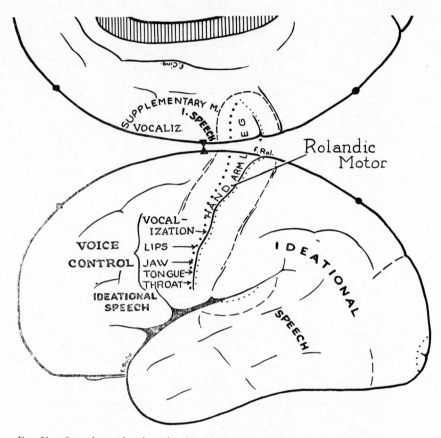

FIG. X-3. Speech mechanisms in the dominant hemisphere. Three areas are devoted to the ideational elaboration of speech; two areas, devoted to vocalization. The principal area devoted to motor control of articulation, or voice control, is located in lower precentral gyrus. Evidence for these localizations is summarized from the analysis of cortical stimulation and cortical excision. See Chapters II, VIII, and IX.

man's ability to talk. Another striking peculiarity of the human motor cortex, which may also bear some relationship to speaking and writing, is the relatively large area devoted to mouth, as indicated in Figure X-3, and the relatively large area for hand as well. It is evident, also, that cortical control of the voice, including articulatory movements and vocalization, is located between the two principal areas for ideational speech, one posterior and the other anterior (see Fig. X-4). The homologous area for voice control on the non-dominant side is shown in Figure X-13.

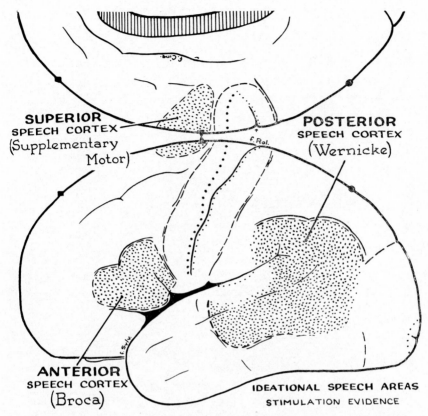

SUPERIOR
SPEECH CORTEX
(Supplementary
Motor)

POSTERIOR
SPEECH CORTEX
(Wernicke)

ANTERIOR
SPEECH CORTEX
(Broca)

IDEATIONAL SPEECH AREAS
STIMULATION EVIDENCE

FIG. X-4. Summarizing map of the areas of cortex in the dominant hemisphere which are normally devoted to the ideational elaboration of speech. Conclusions derived exclusively from the evidence of electrical speech mapping, as discussed in Chapters VII and VIII. Compare with Figure X-10.

It would appear that these Rolandic areas of voice control can serve the purposes of speech on either side alone. Excision of one of the vocalization areas alone does not interfere permanently with speaking. Removal of the lower Rolandic motor cortex (face, jaws, tongue, and throat) can be carried out on one side without abolishing speaking. It produces dysarthria, thickness of speech, which improves gradually until voice control is normal.

Either one of the *supplementary motor areas* can be removed without producing paralysis of limbs or mouth. In the hemisphere which is dominant for speech this produces aphasia which is of several weeks duration, after which it clears up completely. There remains only some slowness of rapidly alternating movements, especially in the opposite hand or foot.*

Erickson and Woolsey (1951) produced evidence to support our conclusion that local discharge would produce vocalization in the supplementary motor area. Chusid et al. (1954), also Erickson and Woolsey, reported aphasia from pressure on the area. Guidetti (1957) produced vocalization by electrical stimulations of the supplementary motor area and observed aphasia of moderate duration following tumor removal from the area in a series of ten brain tumor cases and one atrophic epileptogenic lesion.

From the point of view of the organization of the ideational speech mechanism it is of interest that we have removed the lower Rolandic motor cortex in the dominant hemisphere without producing aphasia, except as a transient postoperative phenomenon.† This will be discussed below.

2. *Ideational speech mechanisms*

The areas of cortex utilized in the ideational elaboration of speech have been outlined by using the application of a gentle electrical current to the proper areas of the cortex of the dominant hemisphere in conscious human beings. The interfering current causes the patient to become aphasic until the electrode is withdrawn. We have called this "aphasic arrest." See Chapters VII and VIII.

Three areas have been outlined thus, as shown in Figure X-4: a) a large area in the posterior temporal and posterior-inferior parietal regions, b) a small area in the posterior part of the third frontal convolution, anterior to the motor voice control area, and c) part of the supplementary motor area within the mid-sagittal fissure and just anterior to the Rolandic motor foot area. For the sake of brevity they may be referred to as the Posterior, the Anterior, and the Superior Cortical Speech Areas—or as *Wernicke's area, Broca's area*, and the supplementary speech area.

---

* A stenographer observed, more than a year after such a removal, that she was slow with the up and down finger movements of the opposite hand in typing, and perhaps of both hands. Another patient observed that following operation she continued to be slow in shaking the opposite foot to get the snow off her boot in winter time.

† It is our impression that excision of the motor-speech area on the left produces anarthria that is more severe and more persistent than on the non-dominant side. But the number of cases in which this has been carried out is not great enough to be statistically significant.

The *supplementary speech area* is the most easily dispensable: The evidence derived from cortical ablations in the dominant hemisphere indicates that removal of the supplementary area produces an aphasia that disappears within a few weeks (Chapter IX).

Broca's speech area is more nearly indispensable than the supplementary area, but our evidence leads us to believe that Marie was probably correct when he asserted that this area of cortex could be sacrificed without eventual loss of normal speech in the adult. Burckhardt (1891) made the same claim, and Mettler (1949) and Jefferson (1950) have agreed from widely different evidence.

Perhaps it is better to express the situation as follows: After destruction of Broca's area the resultant aphasia has eventually cleared up completely in some cases. But the evidence is too meagre to allow one to say all cases, as yet. We have ourselves removed the area in one case of brain tumor only. That patient had an indolent brain tumor classified as hamartoma. But we have never excised it with a simple atrophic lesion in the treatment of focal epilepsy.

On the contrary, in the *posterior speech area* any large destruction that involves cortex and the underlying projection areas of the thalamus would certainly produce the gravest aphasia.

Our conclusion regarding surgical procedures is as follows: Despite the suspicion of dispensability of the anterior speech area of Broca, we still advise that this area, which can be outlined so clearly by stimulation, should be carefully avoided during surgery. No excision should be carried out in the posterior speech area of adults, unless the removal is small.

It is clear that in cases of cortical destruction some degree of displacement of speech function is possible within the same hemisphere. But this substitution of one area for another does not seem to take place when there are continuing local epileptic discharges in the cortex. In some cases removal of epileptogenic cortex may be justifiable, even within the last stronghold of the speech cortex, if that area is invaded by a glioma or if it constitutes an actively discharging epileptogenic focus. The question of displacement of speech function from one hemisphere to the other was discussed in Chapter VI.

In the non-dominant hemisphere the area of cortex which corresponds with the posterior speech area has a function also. Removal produces the syndrome of *apractognosia* (Hécaen, Penfield,

Bertrand, and Malmo, 1956). The patient loses awareness of body-scheme and of the spatial relationships about him (see Fig. X-13).

In conclusion, it is evident that the *motor mechanism for speech* normally depends upon the cortical mechanism for voice control located in the Rolandic motor strip of the two hemispheres (Figs. X-3 and X-13). But if either of these motor areas is destroyed, the other is made in time to do duty for both.

The ideational mechanism of speech is organized for function in one hemisphere only. All three of the cortical areas play roles in this mechanism under normal conditions. When any one of these areas is paralyzed, aphasia results. After removal of the superior speech area there is rapid return of normal speech. After removal of the anterior speech area there is return to normal speech sometimes, possibly always. The posterior speech area is indispensable to normal speech.

In a child a major lesion of the posterior speech cortex, or of the underlying thalamus, would produce transfer of the whole speech mechanism to the opposite hemisphere. When this happens, the organization of speech in the second hemisphere is apparently the same as we have described it above.

Whether or not such a transfer ever occurs successfully for a patient injured in adult life, our own evidence is not sufficient to decide. Others have reported this, years after major injury to the left hemisphere of an adult. This question is discussed at length in Chapter VI. Reorganization and improvement in speech does occur to some extent in the injured dominant hemisphere of a child and of an adult also. This is clear. But we know of no final proof that the ideational mechanisms of speech can be served by the simultaneous use of functional speech areas in the two hemispheres. This would call for an alteration in the mechanism of speech that would be strange indeed.

The posterior speech cortex is adjacent to the *interpretive cortex* (Figs. III-1 and III-2). Indeed, the two areas seem to overlap as judged by the results of stimulation. This is probably not true functionally. No stimulus has ever produced an experiential or interpretive response at the same time with aphasic arrest. And yet the juxtaposition of the two functions, in this area of cerebral cortex that has expanded so greatly in the human brain, may well be significant.

There must be one single functional mechanism within the dominant hemisphere that employs all three cortical speech areas, and it seems likely that a subcortical center plays a most important role in the mechanism.

D. *Subcortical connections*

In Chapter II it was pointed out that the human cortex is made up of numerous functional areas, each of which has its most important connections with areas of gray matter in the brain stem including the thalamus. Thus, each functional area in the more recently evolved cortex makes possible the elaboration of the function of a portion of the older brain. Expressed in another way, the subcortical areas of gray matter, by means of their projection fibers, serve to coordinate and to utilize the functional activities of cortical areas and to integrate that activity with the rest of the brain. Transcortical association tracts are of importance, no doubt, but certainly of less essential importance than *subcortical integration*.

By analogy, we may inquire, therefore, into the subcortical connections of the speech cortex. Figure II-4 shows the parts of the underlying thalamus that are probably projected to the cortex, drawn from the work of Earl Walker (1938b) on the chimpanzee brain. The projections of thalamus to cortex are extrapolated from that animal to man, and Figure II-3 suggests this projection in two dimensions, with certain additions of our own.

It is apparent that the great *posterior speech area* that is mapped out in Figures X-4 and X-10 probably has projection connections with the pulvinar and the nucleus lateralis-posterior of the thalamus (Figs. X-15, X-16, X-17, X-18, X-19, X-20). These cortico-subcortical connections are diagrammed in Figure X-14, taken from the work of Herbert Jasper, who has indicated the back-and-forth connections of the thalamic nucleus lateralis-posterior and the pulvinar with this portion of the cortex—also the two-way connections of the cortex with the centrencephalic system.

Our own cortical mapping, according to the evidence of electrical stimulation (Fig. X-4) and the evidence from neighborhood excisions (Fig. X-10), has been drawn on the face of the hemisphere of the brain. But in order to see how the cortical speech areas were related to the pulvinar and the rest of the thalamus, a slice was cut through them in a normal brain specimen (Fig. X-5) and slanted a little downward from the horizontal plane so as to include pulvinar. The cross-section of the brain which resulted is shown

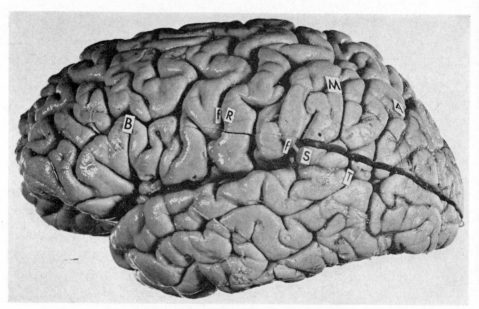

FIG. X-5. Normal brain. B–anterior speech area (Broca), fR–fissure of Rolando, fS-fissure of Sylvius. T–superior temporal fissure, M–supramarginal gyrus, A–angular gyrus. See Figures X-6 and X-7.

in Figure X-6. Broca's convolution is marked B, while the posterior speech area lies well posterior to the fissure of Rolando (fR). A drawing of the photographed cross-section is seen in Fig. X-7.

A second cross-section, 5 mm. above and in a plane parallel to the first, is shown in the photograph, Figure X-8, and a drawing of that cross-section in Figure X-9. These cross-sections show how direct the relationship is. The probable cortical-subcortical inter-relationship of these areas has been shown in diagram (Figs. X-7 and X-9) by the lines which were drawn in with the guidance of our associate, Herbert Jasper. The connections that are indicated by solid lines have been established for the monkey by anatomical studies, and by electrographic recording methods as well. The broken lines of connection to the centrum medianum (C.M.) have been established for the monkey by electrical recording methods only.

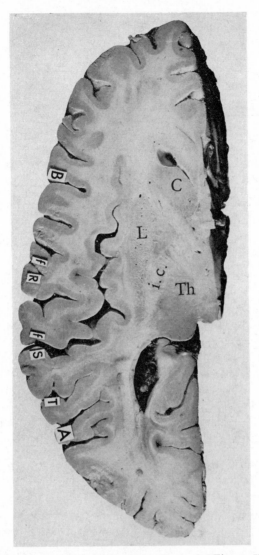

Fɪɢ. X-6. Cross-section of left hemisphere shown in Figure X-5, inclined a little downward so as to pass through pulvinar. Compare with Figure X-7. L–lenticular zone of Marie, C–head of caudate, Th–thalamus.

It is obvious that the connections through pulvinar and centrum medianum (C.M.) make possible a functional inter-relationship between the posterior and the anterior cortical speech areas.

It is proposed, as a *speech hypothesis,* that the functions of all three cortical speech areas in man are coordinated by projections

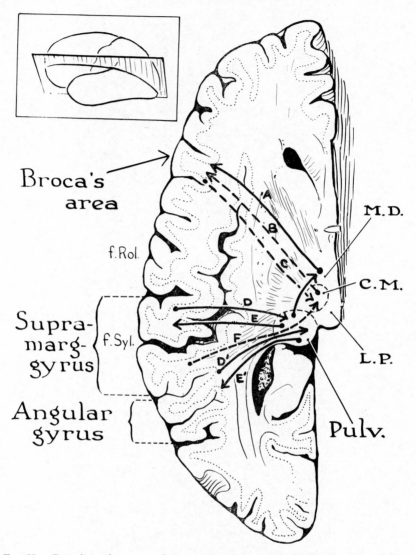

Fig. X-7. Drawing of cross-section seen in photograph in Figure X-6. M.D.–medial dorsal nucleus of thalamus, C.M.–centrum medianum, L.P.–lateral posterior nucleus. See text.

of each to parts of the thalamus, and that by means of these circuits the elaboration of speech is somehow carried out.

Support for such a conception is given by the fact that removal of the gyri all about these two major cortical speech areas does not produce aphasia. Indeed, the map of cortical speech areas shown

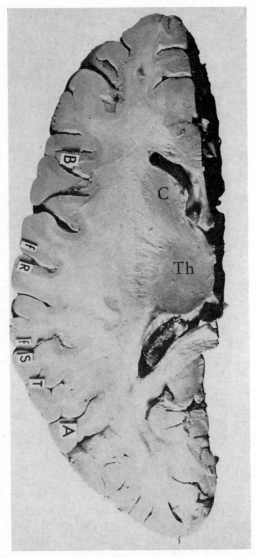

FIG. X-8. Cross-section of left hemisphere 5 mm. above the section shown in Figure X-6. The lettered tickets correspond with those seen on the external surface in Figure X-5.

in Figure X-10 was drawn from the negative evidence provided by successful excisions of gyri close to the speech area, which resulted in no more than transient postoperative aphasia that began several days after operation. Such removals were carried to the bottom of each fissure but never deeper than the gray matter of the gyrus.

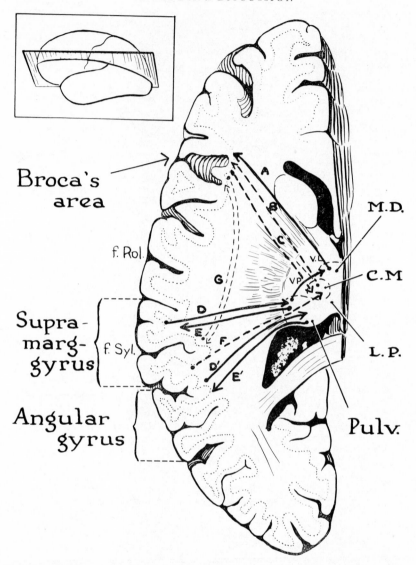

Fig. X-9. Drawing to explain the cross-section seen in Figure X-8. See text.

The removals would not, therefore, interrupt the connections between other gyri and their own subcortical structures under any circumstances. They would also not ordinarily interrupt the more deeply placed transcortical connections in the white matter.

For example: We have removed the visual cortex of the occipital lobe in the dominant hemisphere, and the auditory cortex which covers the transverse gyri of Heschl all the way to the bottom of

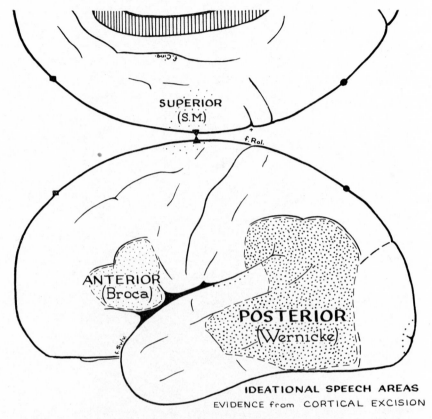

SUPERIOR
(S.M.)

ANTERIOR
(Broca)

POSTERIOR
(Wernicke)

IDEATIONAL SPEECH AREAS
EVIDENCE from CORTICAL EXCISION

FIG. X-10. Summarizing map of the areas of the cortex in the dominant hemisphere which are normally devoted to the ideational elaboration of speech. These conclusions are derived exclusively from the evidence from cortical excisions made around the speech areas (see Chapter IX). Compare with Figure X-4. The size and number of dots used suggests the order of dispensability. Removal of the superior speech area produces aphasia of a few weeks' duration; removal of the anterior area, an aphasia of longer duration.

the fissure of Sylvius, without producing inability to read or to understand spoken speech; we have, several times, removed the lower precentral and postcentral gyrus on either side of the fissure of Rolando at the level shown in the cross-section in Figures X-8 and X-9. This removed the convolutions between the anterior and the posterior speech area. It produced anarthria. There was no aphasia while the patient was on the operating table. Aphasia developed later with the postoperative neuroparalytic edema and cleared up with little delay.

We have removed the anterior 5 or 6 cm. of the left temporal lobe many times, and the cortex of the left insula and the left hippocampal zone as well, without producing aphasia. We have removed the frontal cortex inferior to the Broca's area, as shown in Figure X-10, and the cortex anterior and superior to it as well, without aphasia.

Since all these removals of the convolutions that surround the speech areas do not produce aphasia, it seems reasonable to conclude that the functional integration of these areas must depend upon their connection with some common subcortical zone.

Before continuing the argument it may be useful to consider a vertical cross-section through the pulvinar to compare with Figures X-6 to X-8, which are nearly horizontal. Figures X-11 and X-12

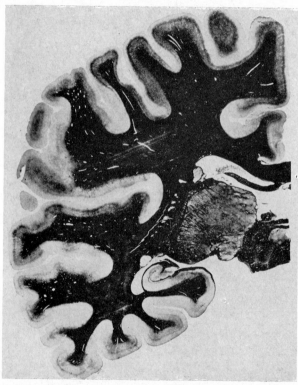

Fig. X-11. Vertical frontal section through the left hemisphere, showing the pulvinar and the fissures of the posterior speech area. Compare with Figure X-12. From Jelgersma.*

* Jelgersma, G. *Atlas anatomicum cerebri humani*. Scheltema and Holkema, Amsterdam.

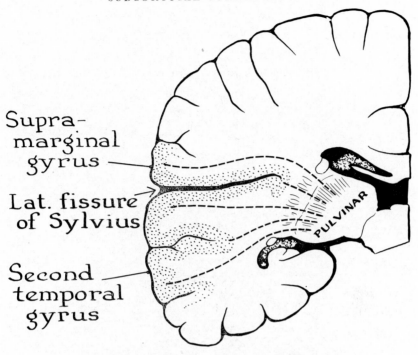

Supra-
marginal
gyrus

Lat. fissure
of Sylvius

Second
temporal
gyrus

SUBCORTICAL PROJECTION
to SPEECH CORTEX

FIG. X-12. Drawing to explain Figure X-11. The hypothetical connections subserving the speech mechanisms are shown by broken lines.

are vertical frontal sections of the left hemisphere taken through the pulvinar, and they show clearly the close relationship of the posterior cortical speech area, with this basal gray nucleus and the adjacent nucleus lateralis-posterior.

These figures also demonstrate the enormous extent of the cortex within these fissures. We have not stimulated the gray matter at the bottom of the fissures to produce aphasic arrest, nor have we ever removed these areas. One can only assume that the convolutions have the same function deep in the fissures as they do on the convexity. The depth of these fissures, as shown in the magnificently stained section from Jelgersma's Human Atlas (Fig. X-11) is truly astonishing.

The drawing by Miss Eleanor Sweezey shown in Figure X-12 explains the preceding Figure. It indicates, also, our interpretation of the functional connection between speech cortex and thalamus.

The broken lines indicate the course of the back-and-forth connection between the pulvinar area and the posterior speech-cortex as mapped out in Figure X-10. The lines drawn in Figures X-7 and X-9 indicate the same to-and-fro connections visualized on a horizontal cross-section.

In the other hemisphere, which is not dominant for speech, this posterior area is devoted to other functional purposes (Fig. X-13). There are no areas for the ideational mechanisms of speech on the non-dominant side, although the motor mechanisms are the same as on the dominant side.

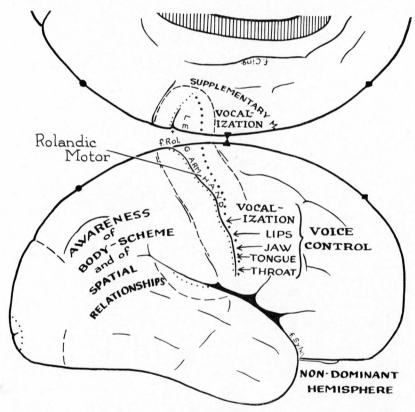

FIG. X-13. Areas devoted to the motor mechanisms of speech in the minor or non-dominant hemisphere. They are similar to those shown for the other side in Figure X-3. Vocalization is produced by stimulation on this side as on the other. A lesion in the voice control area produces dysarthria similarly. Removal of the zone, which would be the posterior cortical speech area of Wernicke in the dominant hemisphere, produces the apractognosic syndrome (Hécaen, Penfield, Bertrand, Malmo, 1956).

It must be assumed, then, that total destruction of the posterior cortical speech area or of the underlying posterior portion of the thalamus would invariably produce global aphasia.

CASE M. St. We have seen a patient recently who had a small hemorrhagic lesion of the pulvinar in the dominant hemisphere without involvement of cerebral cortex. He had severe aphasia. When the disability began to improve, he showed perseveration, he misnamed profusely, and was unaware of his errors.*

But the evidence of the extent of the lesion within the pulvinar depended on clinical examination, arteriography, and ventriculography without autopsy. Therefore, the final proof of extent of lesion is lacking.

Smythe and Stern (1938) reported aphasia in patients who had tumors involving the thalamus alone as determined at autopsy.

When aphasia is produced by electrical stimulation of the anterior or the posterior speech areas of the cortex, it may well be that excitation, extending along the projection fibers from cortex to thalamus, produces functional interference in the thalamus itself, and so results in aphasia. Or the aphasia may be caused simply by the electrical state about the electrode interfering with the use of that area of cortex locally.

A similar type of aphasia is produced when the superior speech area is stimulated, and the aphasic arrest is just as irresistible to the patient as though it were produced in the much more important posterior speech area. This suggests strongly that this superior area also has direct functional connection with some subcortical center, presumably that in the posterior thalamus.

The *aphasia of electrical interference* does not seem to show such variety of pattern as that produced by brain lesions. But this statement may be open to question. The conditions of testing, as described in Chapter V, may explain this apparent sameness. The most frequently used method is the naming of objects shown on cards while the surgeon applies an electric current to the speech cortex at will, here and there. The patient may remain silent, or he may use words to explain that he cannot name the object, or

---

* When shown a pair of scissors, he said, "That is a subscriber." Then he added, "That is an African." A little later he said, "Well, an African knife." When asked if he knew how to use it, he said, "No." But he took up the scissors and used them appropriately. When shown a comb, he said, "That is a symbol." He spelled out the word, symbol, correctly. Then he made a gesture as though to comb his hair,

he may misname it. He may show perseveration. Some would call this *nominal aphasia*. But we have avoided this term since it has been used by neurologists with so many different meanings.

On the basis of the hypothesis that the thalamic center serves in an organizing role, it may be easier to understand the clinical finding that a partial lesion of the posterior speech-cortex produces aphasia which is followed, after a sufficient lapse of time, by recovery without displacement of speech function to the other hemisphere. It makes understandable the recovery of speech function following the aphasia produced by destruction of the superior or anterior cortical speech area. It suggests that the thalamic speech center can be employed for the ideational mechanisms of speech with the assistance of changing (or previously unemployed) areas of the cortex in the same hemisphere.

This speech mechanism which is situated in one hemisphere, combining areas of cortex with a zone of thalamus, must still be integrated into the mechanisms of the whole brain. In Figure X-14 Jasper has indicated the thalamo-cortical connections of the area of cortex on either side. It also shows, in diagram, the "non-specific" connections of cortex and thalamus with the centrencephalic system. This system was described in Chapters II and III as the hypothetical coordinating mechanism that makes possible appropriate employment of various parts of the brain. Thus, the unilateral mechanism of speech must be employed, as needed, in the centrencephalic organization of "travelling potentials" that makes consciousness what it is.

1. *Klingler's cortico-thalamic dissections*

Professor Joseph Klingler of the University of Basel has developed, over the years, a remarkably accurate method of dissecting out the major structures and connections of the brain in fixed specimens. He has described the general results in previous publications. His methods may be found there also (Ludwig and Klingler, 1956).

At our request, Dr. Klingler has made gross demonstrations of the fiber connections that exist between cortex and thalamus, focusing his attention on the areas of cortex which we have described as the posterior, anterior, and superior speech areas (Fig.

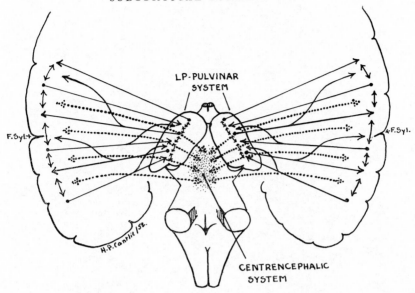

FIG. X-14. Drawing of frontal section through hemispheres and brain stem to show connections of the cortex with pulvinar and with deeper portions of brain stem. Diagrammatic representation of hypothetical thalamocortical relationships of the temporal and parietal cortex with the nucleus lateralis posterior and pulvinar system of the thalamus, and projections (dotted lines) from a centrencephalic system of the brain stem. Drawing by Jasper (Penfield and Jasper, 1954).

X-10). Our general concept of projection connections between the cerebral cortex and the thalamus is illustrated in Figure II-3.

Photographs of the Klingler dissections are presented in Figures X-15, X-17, X-19 and X-21, and following each photograph is a corresponding drawing by Miss Eleanor Sweezey for the purpose of labelling the structures pointed out to her by Dr. Klingler.

The relationship of the posterior speech area of the cortex to the pulvinar is shown by diagram in Figure X-12. The connecting fiber tracts are shown in dissection, as seen from below, in Figures X-15 and X-16, from the lateral side in Figures X-17 and X-18, and from the mesial side in Figures X-19 and X-20.

The cortico-thalamic functional connections that we have proposed are summarized in our diagrams, Figures X-7 and X-9. The dissection seen in Figure X-21 shows the gross connections of Broca's area with the thalamus (dorso-medial nucleus and centrum medianum), explained in Figure X-22. The connection between

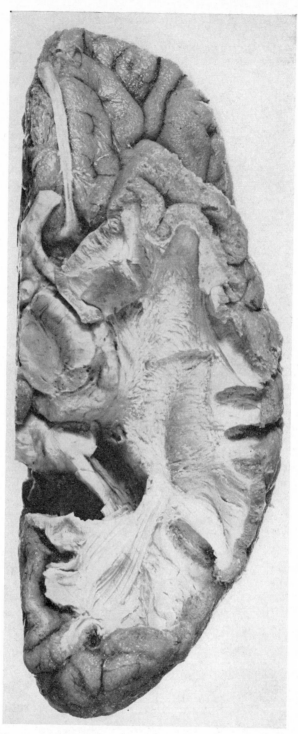

FIG. X-15. Photograph of left hemisphere seen from below to show the nerve fiber projection connections between the posterior speech area on the left middle temporal convolution and the pulvinar. The inferior portion of the left temporal lobe has been removed, together with the inferior horn of the ventricle. Compare with Fig. X-16. Dissection by Professor Klingler.

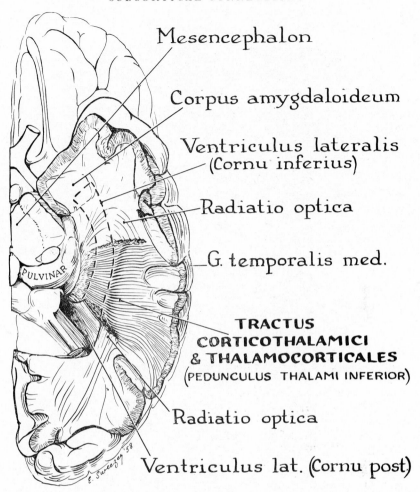

Mesencephalon

Corpus amygdaloideum

Ventriculus lateralis
(Cornu inferius)

Radiatio optica

G. temporalis med.

TRACTUS
CORTICOTHALAMICI
& THALAMOCORTICALES
(PEDUNCULUS THALAMI INFERIOR)

Radiatio optica

Ventriculus lat. (Cornu post)

PULVINAR

FIG. X-16. Drawing of the dissection shown in Figure X-15. The fibers which make up the cortico-thalamic and thalamo-cortical tracts are drawn and labelled.

the cortex of the supplementary motor area and the thalamus is shown in the dissection photographed and drawn in Figures X-19 and X-20.

These gross demonstrations may serve to visualize the general make-up of the speech mechanism as we conceive it in the dominant hemisphere. They present more clearly the anatomical relationships which make our functional hypothesis a plausible one.

219

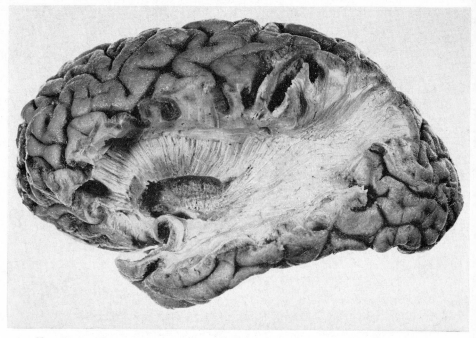

FIG. X-17. Photograph of the lateral surface of the left hemisphere after removal of superficial cortex to show the connecting fibers between the pulvinar and the angular and supramarginal gyri. Compare with Figure X-18. Dissection by Professor Klingler.

E. *Types of aphasia*

Neurologists have long described *aphasia of different types* and their suggestions as to the localization of each major type is summarized, to some extent, in Figure X-1. Some of the most frequent variants of aphasia have been described as follows:

When there was particular difficulty in understanding spoken language, the patient was said to be suffering from 1) *sensory aphasia*. On the other hand, if his major difficulty lay in finding words to express his thoughts, it was called 2) *motor aphasia*; or difficulty in reading, 3) *alexia*; or writing, 4) *agraphia*.

In our own experience, careful testing shows that there are no really pure forms of defect. The patient who has moderate or severe aphasia may be worse in one department of speech. But if he is to be called an aphasic he is rarely, if ever, quite perfect in any department. The differences in the distribution of the de-

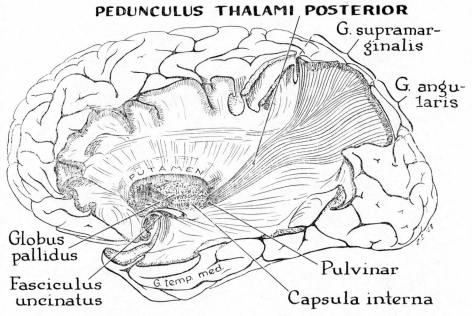

PEDUNCULUS THALAMI POSTERIOR

G. supramar-
ginalis

G. angu-
laris

Globus
pallidus

Fasciculus
uncinatus

G. temp. med.

Pulvinar

Capsula interna

Fig. X-18. Drawing of the dissection shown in Figure X-17 to emphasize the fiber tracts connecting cortex with pulvinar.

fect are important, however, and should, in the end, throw considerable light on the details of function in the speech mechanism.

There are, in the literature of aphasia, many descriptions of *multilingual patients* who have suffered from aphasia affecting one language and not another. We cannot subscribe to the anatomical basis of such a claim. After practicing for thirty years in the bilingual city of Montreal, I have examined many bilingual patients who were said in advance to be aphasic in only one language. In every case, careful testing showed defects in both languages. Emotional factors may influence them in the use of one language rather than the other. But there is no basis for the supposition that one anatomical area of brain is used for one language and a separate area for another. This theme will be elaborated in Chapter XI.

In connection with the varying types of aphasia, the following cases may be of interest. The patients are discussed more fully elsewhere (see the CASE Index).

CASE A. Do. At the time of operation on this patient, the removal bordered on the area marked "writing center" in Figure

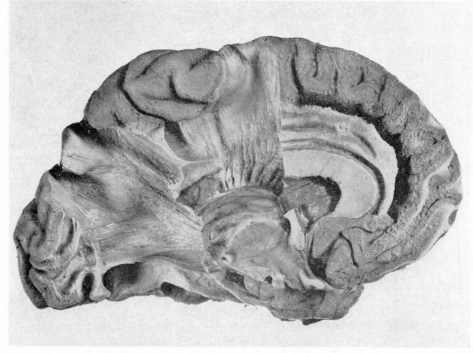

FIG. X-19. Photograph of dissection of the left hemisphere seen from the mesial surface to show the connections between pulvinar and angular gyrus. It also shows the thalamic peduncle (cortico-thalamic and thalamo-cortical tracts) connecting the cortex of the supplementary motor area and the superior speech area with the thalamus. Compare with Figure X-20. Dissection by Professor Klingler.

X-1. Following operation he showed very little evidence of aphasia in superficial conversation, but there was a marked disturbance in ability to write. This cleared up, and three months later he wrote an excellent letter without mistakes.

CASE T. M. We removed the third temporal convolution including the area called by Mills, a *naming center*. After operation the patient showed marked difficulty in naming, but he also had marked interference with writing, reading, and spontaneous speech. Three months after operation this had all cleared up. Careful testing then showed no appreciable difference from his performance before operation.

CASE J. Ma. A small removal carried out in the region of the supramarginal gyrus (Fig. X-2) produced a defect in speech of

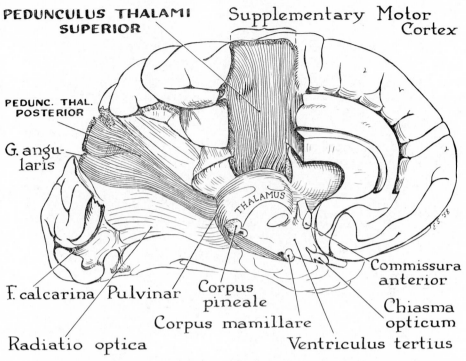

PEDUNCULUS THALAMI SUPERIOR

Supplementary Motor Cortex

PEDUNC. THAL. POSTERIOR

G. angularis

THALAMUS

Commissura anterior

F. calcarina

Pulvinar

Corpus pineale

Corpus mamillare

Chiasma opticum

Ventriculus tertius

Radiatio optica

FIG. X-20. Drawing of the dissection shown in Figure X-19 to show the connections between the posterior speech area of cortex to pulvinar, and similar connections between superior speech area and thalamus.

the type which has been called *word deafness,* a condition which might be described as partial *auditory imperception,* to use Jackson's term. During the postoperative period his aphasia was very severe, due to the removal and to the neuroparalytic edema in adjacent areas. He differed from other patients then and during recovery, because of the severity of his difficulty in understanding spoken words. One year after operation his only defect on testing was a reduced ability to carry out complicated oral commands.

He had, throughout, what many clinicians would have called *sensory aphasia,* and the excision, as well as the neighborhood edema, was in the supramarginal gyrus and first temporal gyrus. This was the area first incriminated by Wernicke.

It was pointed out in Chapter IX that after removal of the motor and sensory face area, the aphasia which resulted brought little interference with understanding of the spoken or written word.

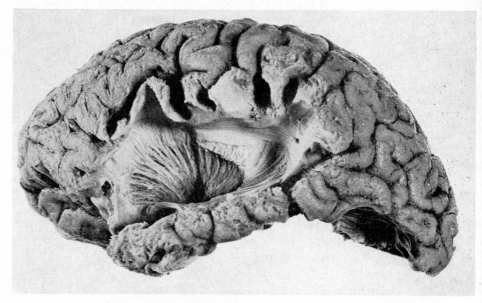

Fig. X-21. Photograph of dissection of the left hemisphere seen from the lateral surface to show connections between thalamus and anterior speech cortex (Broca). Compare with Figure X-22. Dissection by Professor Klingler.

See CASES J. Mo. and W. Pe. But these patients had marked *perseveration* and difficulty in naming, in addition to their dysarthria.

This symptom complex is what clinicians are accustomed to call *motor aphasia*. But in appraising it, the symptoms of anarthria should be clearly distinguished from the aphasic defect.

It should be added that excisions of frontal cortex immediately anterior to Broca's area are followed by aphasia of this motor type. But it has been remarkably transitory, suggesting again that aphasia due to involvement of Broca's area alone is apt not to be severe.

The superior speech area has been excised in a number of instances. The aphasia is of only a few weeks duration. See CASE W. Oe., Chapter IX.

Our experience may be said to support the finding that there is particular difficulty in writing when a lesion is placed in the so-called writing center. The defect is fully recoverable. It supports also the conclusion that the sensory aspects of aphasia are more marked when the lesion is in Wernicke's area, while the motor

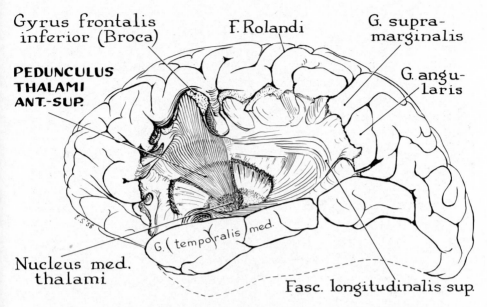

Gyrus frontalis
inferior (Broca)

F. Rolandi

G. supra-
marginalis

PEDUNCULUS
THALAMI
ANT.-SUP.

G. angu-
laris

G. (temporalis) med.

Nucleus med.
thalami

Fasc. longitudinalis sup.

Fig. X-22. Drawing of the dissection shown in Figure X-21. The thalamic peduncle from thalamus to the cortex is clearly shown.

aspects of speech are more damaged by lesions in the general vicinity of Broca's area. But it is evident that the speech mechanism must function as a whole and is not divisible into restricted functional units.

F. *Speaking and thinking*

Up to now we have been discussing localization—seeking the place where speech elaboration dwells. The phrenologists of the 19th century did the same when they palpated the bumps on men's skulls. The only difference was that they were wrong in their conclusions and we are right—we hope! But we will be wrong, too, if we are satisfied to conceive of an independent center for speech acting by itself and let the matter rest there. The phrenologists were more ambitious than we. They sought the hiding place of mother-love, also—and greed, and passion. Thus, they searched for things that have no hiding place. They asked the wrong questions. Scientists, too, may make that mistake, especially today in this era of scientific progress. So many of us load the guns of science and go off hunting for ghosts!

We have been hunting in the field of anatomy and now we must turn toward psychology. Hughlings Jackson (see his Collected Writings, 1931) warned that mixed classifications were dangerous—partly anatomical and partly psychological. For the present we can only conduct parallel lines of argument. And even though they remain parallel and never touch, the findings of functional neuroanatomy may point out a direction for psychological thought.

Jackson ventured far into psychological enquiry, with only his observations of man, in health and disease, for compass. He coined a new word: "verbalizing." Speech, he said, was the second half of the verbalizing process—the second half of a dual process. Perception was the first half, and speaking or the understanding of speech was the second half.

The aphasic patient who tries to speak cannot summon the word symbols of the things he perceives, even though he may summon the images of perceptions. On the other hand, the aphasic who tries in vain to understand speech finds himself unable to carry out the reverse process. He cannot un-verbalize or de-verbalize. In a sense, no doubt, the two defects are similar, because his failure to understand depends upon his inability to utilize the verbalizing mechanism and to summon his own word-images.

But the two cannot have quite identical anatomical mechanisms, for some patients, as already pointed out, have a severe defect in what has been called emitive speech (motor speech) and yet are fairly proficient in receptive or sensory speech, and vice versa.

It is obvious that in many cases the aphasic patient is able to perceive accurately. He knows what an object is used for; he recognizes it. He must, therefore, be able to draw upon his store of recorded experience. He is still able to record his new experience of things heard and seen and to compare the new experience with the whole of his past similar experiences. Thus, his capacity to perceive through other channels than the sound and form of words is preserved.

Wernicke, when he described sensory aphasia in 1874, thought that in the first temporal convolution, next to the area for auditory sensation, there must be a *word-treasury*, "ein Wortschatz;" and near the visual area, a place for "Klangbild," the picture of sound. He was right, in a certain sense. Each of us has a treasury filled with the sounds and the sights of words. But it is clear that the treasury lies in facilitated neurone connections, and in the neurone patterns of the chief cortical speech area of the dominant hemisphere, and in the underlying gray matter of the posterior portions of the thalamus connected with it.

But how do the speech mechanisms work? We have found no "pigeon holes" in the cortex where words are sorted out. Small removals may be made even in the cortex of the posterior speech area, and small injuries may occur there, with eventual recovery after aphasia. And when command of speech returns to the individual, there are no special groups of words to be learned over again, as would be the case if such pigeon holes existed.

For guidance in our psychological enquiry we might well turn back for help to the patient himself whose speech mechanism has been arrested without other obvious interference with thought processes.

CASE C. H. was described earlier (see CASE Index). When the electrode was applied to point 26 (Fig. VII-5, also Frontispiece) on the anterior speech area, the patient was being shown a picture of a human foot. He said, "Oh, I know what it is. That is what you put in your shoes." After the electrode was withdrawn, he said "foot."

When the electrode was applied to the supramarginal gyrus at 27, he said, "I know what it is" and was silent. When the electrode was withdrawn, he said at once, "tree," which was correct.

When the electrode was applied to the posterior temporal region at 28 he was completely silent. A little time after the electrode was withdrawn, he exclaimed suddenly, "Now I can talk—butterfly [which was correct]. I couldn't get that word 'butterfly,' and then I tried to get the word 'moth.' "

This demonstrates that there is a neuronal mechanism for speech in the dominant hemisphere that can be inactivated completely, or incompletely, by electrical interference. Following stimulation at point 28 there was brief epileptic after-discharge, and it seems clear that conduction along the projection fibers to the pulvinar portion of the thalamus must have produced interference there.

The speech mechanism was separately paralyzed, and yet the man can understand what he saw and could substitute the concept, moth, for the concept, butterfly, in a reasoned attempt to regain control of the speech mechanism, by presenting to it a new idea, moth. He could also snap his fingers (as he did) in exasperation at his failure.

The words of C. H. bring us face to face with other *brain mechanisms*. The *concept* of a moth, as distinguished from a butterfly, must also depend on a brain mechanism—a mechanism capable of functioning when the speech mechanism is selectively paralyzed—a mechanism that stores something derived from the past.

A concept, as defined in Webster's Dictionary, is "a mental image of a thing formed by generalization from particulars," and the Oxford Dictionary calls it "an idea of a class of objects."

What C. H. said suggests that an individual normally presents a concept to the speech mechanism and expects an answer. The concept may be butterfly. It may be a person he has known. It may be an animal, a city, a type of action, or a quality. Each concept calls for a name. These names are wanted for what may be a noun or a verb, an adjective or an adverb.

Concepts of this type have been formed gradually over the years, from childhood on. Each time a thing is seen or heard or experienced, the individual has a *perception* of it. A part of that perception comes from his own concomitant interpretation. Each successive perception forms and probably alters the permanent concept. And words are acquired gradually, also, and deposited somehow in the treasure house of word memory—the cortico-thalamic speech mechanisms. Words are often acquired simultaneously with the concepts.

Memory is defined as the power of "reproducing and identifying what has been learned or experienced," (Webster). Memory has many aspects. It requires the employment of more than one mechanism within the brain. There is 1) memory of experiences, 2) memory of concepts, 3) memory of words. Furthermore, there are skills that some might call memories, such as piano playing and driving an automobile. These skills must be different in neuronal organization, and yet they must be mentioned, since they seem to be akin to the skill of writing. Let us consider the first three now:

1) *Experiential memory*. It was pointed out in Chapter III that there is a neuronal record of the stream of consciousness that seems to preserve all those things of which a man was aware, even the unimportant experiences, in a continuous succession from minute to minute to minute. This record of the stream of former consciousness can be activated, occasionally, by electrical stimulation of the interpretive cortex of a conscious man. Under normal conditions the recording mechanism must be called upon subconsciously when a man judges that present experience is familiar or strange, or when he compares the present with past similar experience.

But a man can voluntarily recall the detail of comparatively few past experiences. He can recall the ones that were made memorable because of attendant emotion or because he rehearsed them, immediately afterward and repeatedly, for some reason.

Thus the experiential record serves a man for subconscious interpretations and for the recollection of occasional memorable events.

2) *Conceptual memory*. It is difficult to picture this in the abstract without falling into a confusion of thought. It is simpler to consider a concrete example.

A little boy may first see a butterfly fluttering from flower to flower in a meadow. Later he sees them on the wing or in pictures, many times. On each occasion he adds to his concept of butterfly.

It becomes a generalization from many particulars. He builds up a concept of a butterfly which he can remember and summon at will, although when he comes to manhood, perhaps, he can recollect none of the particular butterflies of past experience.

The same is true of the sequence of sound that makes up a melody. He remembers it after he has forgotten each of the many times he heard, or perhaps sang, or played it. The same is true of colors. He acquires, quite quickly, the concept of lavender, although all the objects on which he saw the color have faded beyond the frontier of voluntary recall. The same is true of the generalization he forms of an acquaintance. Later on he can summon his concept of the individual without recalling their many meetings. When he does so, he expects the man's name to "flash up" in consciousness.

We may compare, now, these two forms of record: the experiential and the conceptual.

Experiential record. When the brain mechanism, that holds the recording of past experience in its patterns of neurone facilitation, is re-awakened by electrical stimulation of the interpretive cortex, the patient might well be aware of a single butterfly in a single meadow. He might hear music, but it would be a specific voice or orchestra making that music as he heard it once in some "forgotten" time. He may see his friend and hear him talk, or he may look at a purple flower. But no generalizations nor concepts are summoned thus.

The conceptual record. Obviously there must be another brain mechanism—one that stores the concepts derived from each series of particulars. This is evidently separate from the experiential mechanism that records the stream of consciousness as described in Chapter III. On the first occasion, when the boy focussed his attention on a butterfly, there was only this particular phenomenon. In it were many particular aspects that he will in time learn to transform into ideas—color, form, movement, beauty. But these characteristics, taken together now, constitute the butterfly.

If the boy's mother was with him when he first paid attention to a butterfly, he probably heard her say the word, "butterfly," and then he said the word himself, as well as he could. In kindergarten later, he would read the word, seeing the picture of a butterfly, and he would write the word, perhaps. Thus he hears, speaks, reads, and writes the new word. He uses a specialized mechanism within the brain to preserve the word with its quadruple aspect. This word mechanism, as we have seen, is localized within the dominant hemisphere.

At the time of the original experience the word was associated with one beautiful object. It delighted him, and that emotion held his attention for the moment. But in time, after more experiences, the first butterfly was forgotten and the word was related to the generalization that he was forming—the concept of a butterfly.

3) *Word memory.* Returning, thus, to speech and the speech mechanism, it is obvious that words which are first related to particulars come to be related to concepts. As time passes there is formed within the brain the *ganglionic equivalent of a word* and the *ganglionic equivalent of a concept.* Experience over the years

continues to reinforce the back-and-forth* neuronal inter-relationship between the two.

Consequently, dropping the terminology of physiology for the moment, I may say that the patient C. H. presented the concept of a "butterfly" to his speech mechanism, expecting that the word for it would be forthcoming. When the mechanism failed him, he cast about and selected an analogous concept from his storehouse of concepts and presented that to the speech mechanism. But again he was disappointed, and he snapped his fingers in exasperation. He could still express himself emotionally with his fingers in that way, although he would probably not have been able to write the lost words.

It is obvious that back-and-forth (or round and round) neuronal conductions between the ganglionic-equivalent of a word and the ganglionic-equivalent of an idea is so facilitated as to be fixed for life. This facilitation is possible, since the nerve cells are quickly habituated to the passage of impulses through a repeated pattern. This aptitude explains the establishment of all *conditioned reflexes*.

So it comes about that as soon as the idea is selected by the individual, the word is normally forthcoming, and the individual, by conscious action, may speak the word, or write the word, or silently formulate the word without external expression. This brings us back to the introductory discussion in Chapter I of what happens in any lecture.

Contrariwise, when an individual is listening or reading, the word immediately summons the corresponding idea. The nerve impulses do not go back along the same fibers but must swing in a circuit to come back to the ganglionic equivalent of a concept, for functional conduction is dromic, i.e. forward, not antidromic or backward.

Three areas of cerebral cortex devoted to ideational speech are indicated in Figure X-4. But electrical stimulation there summons no words. Instead, it throws the whole mechanism out of action. Whether stimulation of the posterior end of the thalamus, as shown in Figure X-7, might summon words is not known. It seems most unlikely. And yet, thoughts or words sometimes are forced

---

* The expression "back-and-forth" is used loosely. I am not suggesting that the same nerve fibers carry effective potentials in both directions.

into a patient's consciousness during the initial stage of an epileptic seizure. And whatever epileptic discharge can do, electrical stimulation may someday do by lucky chance.

The *skill of speaking* and the *skill of writing* depend upon mechanisms within the brain. But it seems obvious that the patterns of those skills are not to be found in the immediate ganglionic structure of the precentral gyrus. The patterns of piano playing or automobile driving that a man "remembers" are not located there either, nor the brush-skill of the artist who has learned to communicate his concepts to others in the language of art.

We have discussed in detail (Chapter II) the motor areas of cortex which are so obviously employed in speaking (Figs. X-3 and X-13). We have outlined the areas of cortex devoted to voluntary movements of the hand (Figs. II-7 and II-10). But these are no more than motor transmitting stations (Fig. II-2). The patterns of neurone potentials that determine the use of the hand in writing and the mouth, throat, and diaphragm in speaking, reach the cortex from the higher brain stem and pass on to the periphery (Figs. II-3 and II-7). But the acquired patterns of all these skills are probably not preserved in the centrencephalic system, and certainly not in the motor cortex.

The awareness, that must be present before speaking and the understanding of speech is made possible, depends upon the passage of neuronal potentials through the multiform circuits of a centrencephalic system. The infinite complexity of that system in the higher brain stem and its connections with the cortex are far beyond our present capacity to visualize.

It is clear that, as the content of the stream of consciousness is never twice the same, so the patterning of centrencephalic organization is always changing. Where, then, are the learned patterns of the various skills—in what ganglionic circuits?

In this monograph it is enough that we should try to answer that question only in regard to the skills of writing and reading. The repository of these skills is clearly in one hemisphere only. It may be that the other skills are served by what are called conditioned reflexes in the two hemispheres.

That the skill of writing depends upon an area of the dominant hemisphere, quite separate from the primary motor mechanisms, is evident from the fact that any man (or child) who loses the right arm can learn to write with the left. He does not have to form new brain patterns for writing. It will not be long before his signature recovers its true character. Then, even the suspicious bank clerk will cash his cheque because the old form of signature returns.

The pattern of the signature and of the writing is in the brain, not in the hand. It is evidently located within the speech mechanism of the dominant hemisphere, and it will serve him, regardless of whether he writes with his right hand, his left hand, or his foot. The same must be true of his speaking, regardless of whether he has his voice control through the cortical motor area in the left hemisphere, the right hemisphere, or both.

Whenever a man speaks or writes, he must first select the concepts that best serve his purpose from a conceptual mechanism. *Conceptual mechanism* seems a better expression than *conceptual store-house,* but neither term should suggest that the place of storing or the manner of activating is understood. Nevertheless, the study of aphasics shows clearly that the speech mechanism is separable from it. This necessitates the hypothesis that there is a conceptual store-house.

One might easily consider that these concepts are preserved somehow in the *centrencephalic system.* But it would seem better to reserve the name centrencephalic for the system which is forever busy with the organization of the present.

Jackson suggested that perception was the second half of the verbalizing process. It would then be the second half when listening and the first half when speaking. To follow his line of thought it would seem that selection of concepts is the first part of the process of writing or speaking, and that the awakening of the individual's own word patterns is the second part. Voluntary use of those patterns to write or to speak is a third part. The act of speaking probably depends upon the functional action of the centrencephalic system. It accepts the word patterns from the speech mechanism and sends out a stream of voluntary impulses through the cortical motor stations of voice control or hand control.

One must suppose, then, that concepts are selected by action of the centrencephalic system, and that the resultant activation of each concept brings up in turn the patterns of corresponding words by *acquired automatic reflex* action. Following this, the centrencephalic system sends forth the patterned stream of impulses that ends in speech or writing.

Reception of speech implies a reverse process: Listening to speech or reading a book would send a stream of afferent impulses flowing inward over the auditory or the visual route, through the transmitting stations of the cortex, into the centrencephalic system. From here the stream must somehow exert its patterned effect upon the speech mechanism of the dominant hemisphere. Ganglionic counterparts of the words are thus activated in the speech mechanism. As each word complex is thus activated, it wakens, by its own automatic reflex, the corresponding concept. Thus, we have come around a circle which depends on the reflex connection of each word or succession of words with each corresponding concept. The connection between *speech mechanism* and *concept mechanism* is evidently reflex and automatic.

Thus, a man listening to a speaker may follow the man's words, ignoring the concepts; or he may attend only to the concepts of which the words are symbols, ignoring the words. If this listener is bilingual, he may fail to notice what language the speaker had used.

In conclusion, the first sure evidence that physicians might hope to distinguish functional units within the brain, appeared about one hundred years ago with the discovery of a speech mechanism within one hemisphere. The purpose of this monograph is to throw new light on that mechanism. In doing so, we have attempted at the same time to set before the reader a simple statement of present evidence in regard to sensory, motor, and psychical functions of the human brain.

Now that we can recognize the parts of dominant cortex and thalamus that are devoted to the learning of speech and to its uses, we must seek constructive hypotheses which fit the function of speech into the total functioning of the brain.

The clinical and physiological observations we have made should serve as permanent building stones. The deductions and hypotheses must face the tests of time. And if they are proven wrong, we may still take comfort in the hope that, before they are discarded, they will have served a useful purpose to explorers who pass this way.

CHAPTER XI

EPILOGUE—THE LEARNING OF LANGUAGES

W. P.

THIS closing chapter is a discussion of language learning. Surely a consideration of the neurophysiological mechanisms of speech should have some educational consequences. This final chapter may therefore interest parents and teachers more than the more technical discussions in the earlier chapters.

A. *From physiology to education*

In 1939 I was asked to give an address at Lower Canada College, and I decided to talk directly to the boys. Excerpts from that talk may serve as an amusing introduction here.

"I have long wondered," my talk began, "about secondary education from the safe distance of a neurological clinic. I have wondered why the curriculum was not adjusted to the evolution of functional capacity in the brain . . .

"Before the age of nine to twelve, a child is a specialist in learning to speak. At that age he can learn two or three languages as easily as one. It has been said that an Anglo-Saxon cannot learn other languages well. That is only because, as he grows up, he becomes a stiff and resistant individualist, like a tree—a sort of oak that cannot be bent in any graceful manner. But the Anglo-Saxon, if caught young enough, is as plastic and as good a linguist as the child of any other race.

"When you have graduated and have left Lower Canada College behind you, I hope that some of you will go into teaching as a profession, for there is no more important, no more challenging, and no more enjoyable profession than that of a teacher. But when you enter that profession, I beg you to rearrange the curriculum according to the changing mental capacities of the boys and girls you have to teach. . . . Remember that for the purposes of learning languages, the human brain becomes progressively stiff and rigid after the age of nine."

At the close of that somewhat naive address the boys and their parents seemed most enthusiastic. What the teachers thought is not difficult to imagine. At all events, they smiled politely.

Again in 1953 I was called upon to address a lay audience. It was at a meeting of the American Academy of Arts and Sciences in Boston. By that time Dr. Roberts and I were in the midst of our clinical studies of speech disorders. Consequently, I chose as my subject: "A consideration of the neurophysiological mechanisms of speech and some educational consequences" (Penfield, 1953).

This aroused far more interest than I could have anticipated. The officers of the Modern Language Association of America heard of it, and, probably because it coincided with their own views, they had it reprinted. It was distributed then to the far flung membership of that Association.

This dissemination resulted in at least one adverse criticism. A university president objected that early teaching of secondary languages was somehow in opposition to the teaching of those languages in institutions of higher learning. My intention, however, had been to promote more and better work in modern languages at the university level. But I consoled myself with the thought that there was, after all, nothing new in my proposals. Indeed, the ideas put forward were considerably older than modern education.

The world seems to have grown so much smaller and its peoples, all around the world, feel the need of direct communication. It is this need that emboldens us to add this chapter, which is primarily a scientific enquiry into *language learning*, and secondarily a plea for more consideration of the significance of neurophysiology in education.

It may well be convenient, for those who must plan the curriculum, to postpone the teaching of secondary languages until the second decade of childhood. But if the plan does not succeed, as they would have it, let them consider whether they have consulted the time table of the cerebral hemispheres. There is a biological clock of the brain as well as of the body glands of children.

Suppose a government, anxious about over-population, were to pass a law that marriage must wait until the age of forty. Perhaps there might be certain advantages for such a plan! Perhaps the plan might prove to be wise, too, if men and women were machines instead of the living, growing, changing creatures that they are. Such a law, you may well say, would be contrary to the unfolding nature of men and women. But, the same is true of a school curriculum in which the teaching of secondary language makes its first appearance at twelve or sixteen years of age.

For *bilingual countries* like Canada and Belgium, and for *multilingual countries* like India and the U.S.S.R., the learning of secondary languages is of the greatest importance. But unilingual lands have no less need of learning secondary languages. Ignorance deafens us so we cannot hear what our brothers are saying in other lands. Ignorance also blinds us so we cannot see them.

B. *A glance backward and downward*

In the *history* of the human race we can only surmise how it was that man began to speak. Bees have a way of communicating ideas. So do birds and dogs and monkeys. They communicate ideas without words or names. The brain of the dog resembles the human brain in general organization. The brain of the chimpanzee is even more like ours. All the lobes are present. The pathways of muscular control are similar. Chimpanzee and dog have large areas of cerebral cortex, like our own, used for seeing, hearing, feeling. They have even larger areas for smelling.

More than that, animals have in their brains a mysterious store of useful instincts that I like to consider racial memories. These racial memories guide them at crucial times in life—teach them how to build a home and what to hunt. Man's brain is curiously lacking in these patterns of instinctive guidance for his behavior.

But to balance all that, man has the ability to learn. He is teachable. The infant possesses a *speech mechanism*, but it is only a potential mechanism. It is a clean slate, waiting for what that infant is to hear and see. Language must be taught first. And then, in time, language will serve as the vehicle for practically all forms of knowledge.

In the beginning, before he speaks, a child learns to know the meaning of the objects about him. Animals do the same. He understands certain concepts such as going out of doors, eating, etc., from experience. Animals do the same. He learns to understand the names for simple concepts, and animals follow him there, too, a little way.

When the child begins to speak, the animal is blocked and can no longer follow. This may be explained in part, perhaps, by the fact that man alone has an inborn control mechanism for vocalization in his cerebral cortex (see Fig. X-3). Animals bark or mew or chatter by using neurological motor mechanisms in what may be called the old brain. Without the help of man's vocalization projection to the newer cortex, it is quite possible that vocalization could not be used in the complicated patterns which he employs for human speech. This must remain an hypothesis.

However, the neurological structures required for another and much more important mechanism are probably missing, too, in the subhuman brain. That is the mechanism employed by man for ideational speech. There is a very large increase in the extent of the temporo-parietal cortex that becomes obvious in passing from anthropoid ape to man. It seems likely that the posterior speech area of the human cortex (Fig. X-10) constitutes a new appearance. It might seem that, by its addition, it had pushed the sensory and motor areas away and down into the fissures, and so, taken over this zone as the major ideational speech structure. One may assume that when these evolutionary enlargements of the brain made their appearance, in a far off time, man began to talk. This, too, is hypothesis.

Reference to Figures X-3 and X-4 shows that the posterior speech area is the largest. It is clearly the most important and the most indispensable area. It is not clear why there should be a second anterior and a third superior area devoted to speech. But nature has done a similar thing in regard to the cortical motor area (see Fig. II-10). There is a primary motor area on the precentral gyrus and a separate supplementary motor area. There are also primary and secondary sensory areas, as shown in that figure.

The appearance of *writing* is certainly a much more recent event. This is even within the most distant limits of history. Collective civilization seems to have been made possible when man learned to cultivate grain in the valleys of the Nile and the Euphrates.

At the Iraq Museum in Baghdad is to be seen a most exciting series of clay tablets unearthed from ancient Sumerian cities where the Euphrates and Tigris rivers flowed into the Persian Gulf. These clay tablets are shaped like pieces of soap. At the time of writing, the tablet of soft clay was held in the palm of one hand while the scribe printed the cuneiform letters onto its surface, using a sharp stylus held in the other hand.

Many stages in the evolution of writing, beginning some 5,000 years ago, are to be seen in Baghdad.* One of the earliest tablets shows a pictograph of a bag of barley, and following it from left to right, suggesting that the scribe was holding the stylus in his right hand, is the single mark of the stylus that stood for the number ten (the number of a man's fingers). That is followed in turn by the marks to signify ones.

This was a record of sale at a time when speech must have been well advanced. It was a time when men were about to turn from the use of pictographs to writing. The development of their cuneiform writing from that time onward seems to have been relatively rapid.

C. *The direct method of language learning*

The learning of language in the home takes place in familiar stages which are dependent upon the evolution of the child's

---

* I was indebted to Seton Lloyd, who was Curator of the Iraq Museum in 1943 at the time of my first visit, for the demonstration of these tablets. Somewhat similar tablets may be seen also in the museum of the University of Pennsylvania in Philadelphia, and in the British Museum in London.

brain. The mother helps, but initiative comes from the growing youngster. The learning of the mother tongue is normally an inevitable process. No parent could prevent it unless he placed his child in solitary confinement!

The learning of language by the direct method (the mother's method) is far more successful than the school-time learning of secondary languages in the second decade of life (*language education*). The reasons for the success of the first method may be considered under two headings: 1) Physiological, and 2) Psychological.

1. *Neurophysiology.* The physiological reason for success in the home is that a child's brain has a specialized capacity for learning language—a capacity that decreases with the passage of years.

Evidence for this may be found in the experience of any immigrant family that arrives in a new country without previous knowledge of the local language. In two years the children learn a new language. They may come to speak it easily, with little accent, regardless of whether they go to school or simply play in the street. The same cannot be said of their parents. They seem to have lost the art of learning by a direct method. They may have recourse to special teaching by the scholastic or indirect method, but they cannot compete with their children. Their learning is indirect because they use the units of the mother tongue, which I shall describe below.

The brain of the child is plastic. The brain of the adult, however effective it may be in other directions, is usually inferior to that of the child as far as language is concerned. This is borne out still further by the remarkable re-learning of a child after injury or disease destroys the speech areas in the dominant left cerebral hemisphere (see Chapter VI). Child and adult, alike, become speechless after such an injury, but the child will speak again, and does so, normally, after a period of months. The adult may or may not do so, depending on the severity of the injury.

Examples of completely successful transfer of speech mechanism from the left to the right hemisphere in children under three or four years of age are numerous. The upper age limit for this is not certain. But when the injury to the dominant hemisphere of an adult in his twenties or beyond is severe enough, he may never recover normal speech.

It must not be assumed, of course that speech is the only new skill that is more rapidly and perfectly acquired in childhood than it is later. Perhaps piano and violin playing and skiing come into similar categories.

2. *Psychology.* The second reason for the success of the direct method of teaching language in the home is the *psychological urge.* This must not be overlooked. For the child at home, the learning of language is a method of learning about life, a means of getting what he wants, a way of satisfying the unquenchable curiosity that burns in him almost from the beginning. He is hardly aware of the fact that he is learning language, and it does not form his primary conscious goal.

The same may be true of a young child who is learning a new language in school, but it is only true if no other language is being spoken, for the time being, in the class room. The direct method is then employed in school, but the impetus for learning should still not be to collect words nor to acquire language. It should be to achieve success in games and problems, and success in learning about life and other delightful things.

It is interesting to speculate as to how such a man as William Shakespeare learned the English language. It seems quite unlikely that his mother could have taught him grammar or syntax, and one may doubt that such teaching in school was in any way responsible for the great gift of expression that was his, and the vast store of words in his memory. He must have learned English by the direct method at home, like other children. And, as he passed out of the primary stage of language learning into the second stage of *vocabulary expansion* in school, his rapid brain embraced thousands of new words in yearly succession.

The direct method of learning language can succeed at an older age—even after nine years—and adults can, of course, learn by it. The success of the Berlitz method is evidence of this. Some adults do quite well.

Take the case of Josef Konrad Korzeniowski, a Polish boy born in the Ukraine. He also became a master of the English language, second only to Shakespeare, perhaps. As a British subject and a celebrated author he was known as Joseph Conrad. English was for him a secondary, or rather, a tertiary language. Polish was his mother's tongue, but he spoke French as a child with his nursery governess, and he sailed away on a British ship at the age of fifteen years.

At sea he heard no other language but English, and so, at fifteen he began to learn this language by the "mother's method." He learned the "lingo" and the slang first, no doubt. The *psychology of language learning* in this sailing ship was like that in the home. There was no translating. English words were the immediate symbols through which he must come to understand life. They were the symbols that brought him food and success as a young sailor.

Thus, he learned the sort of language he would never have discovered, however hard he worked, with dictionary and grammar as his only guide. He learned the good, short, simple words and the speech that men use in the face of trial and danger.

"Goodbye brothers," he wrote, "you were a good crowd. As good a crowd as ever fisted with wild cries the beating canvas of a heavy foresail; or tossing aloft, invisible in the night, gave back yell for yell to a westerly gale."

I have been told by an Englishman, who knew Conrad after he had become a famous author in England, that he spoke English beautifully. He recalls, now, no obvious accent, either Polish or French. I suspect, however, that his accent at first and his early vocabulary must have resembled to some extent that of the sailors with whom he shipped. But once he had mastered the elements of that limited shipboard vocabulary in English by the direct method, he was ready to expand his English vocabulary in any and all directions.

There is some evidence to suggest that those who learn more than one language in early childhood find the learning of later additional languages easier. Theoretically it should be so, since they carry in their speech mechanism a larger variety of sound elements and speech units. I shall enlarge on this presently.

D. *The biological time-table of language learning*

The sequence of normal language learning has been studied exhaustively by Leopold (1939-49) in his own children, who were brought up in a bilingual household, and by Gesell and Ilg in a large series of unilingual children, followed through succeeding years.*

During the infant's first year he cries at once. He coos later and then babbles. Babbling is verbal play "with front sounds and clear consonants." Around the time of the first birthday he usually says his first word. In the second year it is clear that the child learns to understand and later to speak. There is apt to be a lag of 2 to 7 months from first hearing to utterance. From 2 to 4 years the delightful lingo of baby talk disappears and is replaced by adult pronunciation. The skills of understanding and speaking are more or less perfected by the age of 4. Reading and writing are not yet to be considered.

Leopold concludes that during the second year of life speech consists normally of one-word sentences. Gradually the child puts two words together, then three. There are many variations to these achievements, as any proud parent will testify. But by the time of the third birthday the three basic elements of simple sentences have made their appearance: subject, verb, object. The child uses some pronouns and employs plurals at this time, and is adding new words at the rate of about four hundred in six months.

Dr. Ilg would distinguish two types of child, which she calls "imitative" and "creative." Children in the first group learn more rapidly and accurately with less baby talk and jargon. Girls are more likely to be placed in this group of accurate learners than boys. The creative learner is slower and more apt to elaborate pronunciations and jargon of his own. Poets, she says, are prone to come from this group! It is obvious that individual differences are recognizable at almost any stage throughout childhood.

There seems to be little if any relationship between general intellectual capacity and the ability of a child to imitate an accent. Pronunciation is essentially an imitative process. Capacity for imitation is maximum between 4 and 8. It steadily decreases throughout later childhood.

According to Professor Leopold the child of 6 to 8 years has formed his native speech habits completely. But they are not so firmly established as to interfere with his capacity to acquire a second language without translation. It would seem, however, that the

* See also *Bulletin No. 49*, August 1956, issued by the Modern Language Association of America, 6 Washington Square, North, New York 3, N.Y.

first language is well set by the age of 4 or 5. As I shall point out later, if the child is using a second language even before that time, the two may be set equally without interference.

Gesell and Ilg have concluded that at the age of 8 the average child is "group-minded, expansive and receptive." At 8 the child begins to hold on to patterns, and at 9, to fix these patterns. At the age of 9 the child is said to become more analytical in language learning. He is apt to become analytical in regard to his general attitude as well.

E. *Brain-mechanisms of language*

Man's ability to talk is due to the development and employment of the specialized speech mechanisms of the dominant hemisphere, as described in the preceding chapter. Local injury of these areas in early childhood may produce a complete aphasia. This is followed by a period of silence, to be succeeded in time by complete re-learning of language. The ability of an adult to re-learn speech after injury is much inferior to that of a child.

With severe aphasia at any time, the individual's ability to convey meaning by gesture of head or hand is lost. He may use the muscles of neck and hand for other purposes, but he cannot nod assent in place of the word "yes," nor shake his head in place of the lost word "no." It must be assumed, then, that the characteristic gestures employed by anyone to convey meaning while speaking, or instead of speaking, must have neuronal units in the speech mechanism. This applies to meaningful gestures as it does to writing.

No statement of the evidence in regard to speech dominance and hand dominance need be made here.* As far as our evidence can go, grave injury in infancy or childhood produces transfer of speech dominance to the opposite hemisphere, if the lesion occurs in the speech area. But hand dominance is not caused to change over unless there is injury to arm areas also. Thus the transfers are independent.

However, since injuries are apt to involve both areas rather than one, it can be understood that an individual who is left-handed because of early disease or brain injury is most likely to have

* The reader has only to turn to Dr. Roberts' exhaustive study in Chapter VI.

speech function located in the right hemisphere. On the other hand, the "normally" left-handed individual who had no early brain injury may have speech dominance in either hemisphere. But he is still more apt to have it in the left hemisphere like other people.

It seems unlikely that speech correction or speech development can be aided by interference with the spontaneous tendency to use right or left hand in preference. It is also impossible for the observer to be certain (unless a radical sodium amytal aphasia test is carried out) whether, during the period of recovery from aphasia, the individual is making a transfer of speech function to the opposite hemisphere, as children sometimes do, or whether he is restoring function in the injured hemisphere, as adults are more likely to do.

Now to return to the normal process of language learning: The cerebral mechanisms involved in learning a language by the direct method may be pictured in hypothetical outline. For clarification and a statement of the evidence, the reader may turn to Chapter X, and especially to the final section F. on "Speaking and Thinking."

1. *Acquisition of speech units.* Consider the second year of a child's life. The opinion of Leopold was quoted above, that at this age there is a lag of two to seven months from the first hearing of a word until its first meaningful utterance. During that time the child is faced with the necessity of making a neuronal record of the concept to be named and a neuronal record of the word. There is a third task, too. That is to establish an automatic reflex connection between the two.

For example, suppose that each time the mother takes the child out of doors, she says, "Go bye-bye." The child must learn to understand the meaning of the concept of going out of doors. To do that he must make a generalization from a number of particular experiences of going out in his carriage.

That concept must be recorded somewhere in the brain so he can get at it again when needed. It must be held there so he can alter it as time passes and new experiences come to him. One must assume that there are specialized areas in the brain where the patterns of passage of nerve impulse may be stored. The pattern of passage of electrical potentials through certain neurones (nerve cells) and over their connecting fibers forms a unit. In this case the unit becomes the concept (going out of doors) when nerve impulses pass through that pattern again.

Each passage of a stream of neuronal impulses leaves behind it a persisting facilitation, so that impulses may pass that way again with greater ease. This is, in general, the neuronal basis of memory. The pattern followed by those impulses may be referred to as a unit, for the purposes of our discussion. And I shall use the word "unit" to refer to the neuronal pattern that corresponds with the sound of a word. I shall use the word "unit," too, when referring to the neuronal pattern used in speaking the word.

It was pointed out in Chapter X that memory of concepts, which does not depend on one hemisphere as speech does, is separate from the speech mechanism. Conceptual memory may be intact in the presence of severe aphasia when the left-sided speech mechanism is paralyzed. Therefore, a neurone-connection pattern must be established in what may be called the *concept mechanism*. In the case of the child, the idea of going out of doors is preserved as a *conceptual unit.*

In addition, then, to the idea of going out of doors, the child must remember the sound of the words "Go bye-bye." That means that a neurone-connection pattern is laid down in the speech areas of the left hemisphere. This we might call the *sound unit.* In addition to that, there must be an automatic connection from sound unit to conceptual unit, and from conceptual unit to sound unit.

When these two units are established with their interconnections, the baby is able to understand. An intelligent dog might achieve all of these things, too, as far as this process has gone. Now that the baby understands, he probably smiles or laughs at the phrase "Go bye-bye." The dog might well wag his tail under the same circumstances. Each would thus indicate his understanding without speech and add his approbation. It would be communication without words.

But the baby must now take the next step, and no animal can follow him there. He must speak. When he does do so, he will imitate the sound in a voluntary act, probably making one word of it—perhaps something like "bye-bye."

Having spoken, he will repeat that word often. Each time he hears his mother say it in the next few months, he will probably pronounce it better and so make for himself a more and more perfect verbal motor image. This *verbal unit* has its neuronal pattern located in the left hemisphere speech mechanism (Fig. X-10). Certainly, at all events, it is not in the areas of cortex concerned with voice control (Figs. X-3 and X-13), although these motor areas of the cortex must be used in the voluntary formation of the sounds.

What the relationship may be between the word-sound-unit and the verbal-unit is not clear. The verbal-unit seems to formulate for the child the set of the muscles to be used to pronounce the word. Some light may be thrown on this question by reconsidering the types of clinical aphasia.

It was pointed out in Chapter X that there are definite differences in the types of aphasia produced by lesions in different portions of the speech cortex. In some cases there is more involvement of the sensory side of speech, and in others, more of the motor elements. Thus, there is what clinicians have called *motor aphasia*, in which speaking is severely involved while understanding of speech is relatively, and comparatively, intact. There is also *sensory aphasia* in which the reverse is true. This strongly suggests that the motor units for words and phrases are separated somehow, spatially, from the sensory units. But it is also clear that they are both located in the general region of the cortico-thalamic speech areas of the left side, where they are closely interrelated in function.

Thus, when the child begins to understand, he is establishing general concept-units in the brain and corresponding word-sound-units. When he begins to speak he must establish word-formation-units. During this early experimental period he uses his voluntary motor system to make a more and more accurate sound, thus correcting and reinforcing the image of how to speak the word. What I called an image is really a pattern of the motor complex required to produce the word. This image or motor pattern is a unit, too, and the neurones involved in the pattern-unit are clearly located in the speech areas.

Between the motor-pattern-unit and the motor-expression-mechanism the connection is not automatic. If it were, the child would be an automaton, a machine, a robot. No. Between word-pattern and word-expression must come a conscious selection and decision. This means the employment of the *centrencephalic system*. That is the system of central organizing connections which makes available to conscious thinking the many different neuronal mechanisms within the brain. See Chapters I and III.

When the child begins to write words and to read words, two new sets of units must be established. They are also located within the general structure of the dominant hemisphere speech mechanism.

Writing is carried out by one hand, which is called dominant. It is controlled through the motor hand mechanism in the cortex of the opposite hemisphere (Figs. II-2, II-7, II-10). Writing must be considered voluntary in regard to each move, at the beginning. But in time it comes to be automatic. The image of the movement required to produce each word, taken together with the execution of the movement, becomes a skill that is eventually automatic but can be controlled voluntarily. It is so automatic that in time, a man can summon a word and discover that his hand has written it. He can go beyond that. He can summon to mind the concept, of which the word is a counterpart, and discover that his hand has written it. He can summon a series of concepts and find them recorded by that hand on the page before him. Writing, thus, takes on an automatic character like speaking and automobile driving.

The driver of a car makes each move under voluntary control while learning. Later on he thinks only of turning the automobile around the corner, and his hands "do the trick" automatically. Speaking becomes similarly automatic. A man may summon a word and his lips speak it. He may summon a series of concepts and the words are produced automatically.

But, nevertheless, the patterns of how the words are to be spoken and the patterns of the words to be written are each recorded in the speech mechanism, not in the motor mechanism of the right hand. If I should break my right arm and then train my left to do what I want it to do, my signature will soon be accepted by the experts at the bank who knew my name on cheques (all too well!) before the accident.

Let me recall the case of a patient who made his living by his hand writing. He suffered from writer's cramp, and so he had to shift from right hand to left hand, back and forth, because the cramp would come upon him after a few weeks or months. When

I asked him about his signature on cheques, he replied, "Oh, the signature is in the mind."

Yes, he was correct in thinking that the signature was not in the motor mechanism. It is in the neurone unit within the brain. Probably that applies to all the words we write. It seems likely that we write according to the concept carried in the brain. The signature follows that neurone pattern. The written word is carried as a final pattern—a pattern of a motor complex. In the fully developed skill the unit-pattern is only one station in the amazing automatic flow of electrical potentials from concept unit to muscle.

Returning to the act of speaking: We control voice and mouth by following the verbal motor units formed and fixed by early practice. It is difficult to make any certain statement on the question of accents by reference to the physiological evidence alone. One may say that children have a greater capacity for imitation than adults. That seems to be a fact, but it is not an explanation of what happens in later life.

We may reconsider the whole process more simply: During normal speech it may be said that two mechanisms are employed, and both are present only in the human brain. There is an ideational mechanism which makes available the acquired elements of speech, and a motor articulation mechanism that is inborn but may be utilized by the voluntary motor system.

a) The ideational part of speech, whether spoken, heard, written, or read, depends upon the employment of a certain portion of one hemisphere alone—normally the left hemisphere. This localization of a function in one hemisphere is, in itself, something new in mammalian evolution. Other intellectual functions, such as perception, the recording of current experiences, and the storing of generalizations or concepts in memory, are made possible by the utilization of homologous areas of cerebral cortex on the two sides, together with the coordinating and integrating work of the higher brain stem.

It is thanks to the action of the ideational speech areas of the dominant cortex, and their connections with a small zone of gray matter below the cortex in the thalamus, that words may be "found" by the individual. Speech is made possible because of neurone patterns and reflexes that are formed there during the process of language learning.

The nerve cells and nerve branches of some parts of the brain, or perhaps the synapses which join the branch of one cell to the body of another cell, are altered by the passage of a stream of electrical potentials. This is what makes permanent patterns possible. This is the basis of all *memory*.

Thus, man is able to find, in his ideational speech mechanism, four sets of neurone patterns: the sound units of words employed when listening to speech, the verbal units followed for speaking, the visual units for reading, and the manual units for writing.*

This is, no doubt, an oversimplification. And yet it must be somehow true, since other areas of the cortex may be removed without producing aphasia, if only the speech areas of the dominant cortex and its subcortical connections are not interfered with. On the other hand, when they alone are involved, and the rest of the hemisphere is normal, the patient can no longer "find" words, though he "knows" what he wants to say. He can summon the concepts "to mind," but the previously automatic connection between concept unit and word unit is broken. This is *aphasia*.

b) *Articulation*, on the other hand, depends upon the employment of special motor areas in the cortex of either hemisphere. There are areas devoted to vocalization—two in each cortex—and no other mammal yet studied possesses such areas in the motor cortex. There are areas also for other movements of mouth, tongue, and throat.

The streams of neurone impulses that produce voluntary movement arise in the circuits of integration in the brain stem—the *centrencephalic system*. They flow out to these cortical motor areas and from there down to the muscles of mouth and throat and diaphragm. But if the motor areas of cortex are damaged or removed on one side, those on the other side soon serve the purposes of speech movements quite satisfactorily.

Man has inherited the motor mechanisms which make speaking possible. But there is no inheritance of those things that he adds to his ideational speech mechanism while he is learning a language.

---

* It might be suggested that a word or a phrase is sometimes used in thinking without reference to sound of the word, its appearance when printed, or the movements of mouth or hand which make it. This implies that there is an abstract concept of a word. Butterfly is a word. The idea of the fluttering, living thing is a concept. Whether there is something else between the two is a matter for psychological discussion and need not detain us here.

The clean blank speech slate which he brought with him into the world is soon filled with units, and after the first decade of life they can hardly be erased. They can be added to, but with increasing difficulty.

2. *Vocabulary expansion.* When a child comes to the age of 6 he is ready to begin to expand his vocabulary rapidly, and as he passes the age of 9, the process is accelerated. He reads and talks and listens incessantly. If he is expanding his vocabulary in his native tongue, the process is simple, rapid, normal. He uses the speech units already written indelibly on the slate of his ideational speech mechanism.

He can pass from a vocabulary of 1,000 words to 10,000 perhaps, using the same language set. The sound, the pronunciation, and the spelling are all so similar. He can use his recorded units. The sentence construction does not alter. His eventual accent continues to resemble the accent of those he listened to first in home and school and playground.

F. *Second languages*

If the child uses only one language until he becomes a young adult, he then approaches a second language by using the well learned symbols of his mother tongue. This is correct for language-expansion, but wrong for new-unit formation. Instead of imitating the sounds of the new language, he tries to employ his own verbal units—his mother-tongue units—and so, speaks with an accent, and even rearranges the new words into a construction that is wrong. Thus, all Swedes speak English with a Swedish accent, and the French, the Germans, and the Chinese each speak it with their own accents.

This is a common enough experience. Even though they travel over the world, the Cockney and the Scot and the Irishman betray their origin all through life by a "turn of the tongue" learned in childhood, to say nothing of the Canadian and the American.

1. *Language learning by the indirect method.* The youth who approaches a second language for the first time in school, during the second or third decade of his life, faces a new problem. He has come, now, into the period of rapid vocabulary expansion, as well as the period of mathematical, historical, scientific, and philosophi-

cal studies. He employs the units which were fixed in his speech mechanism in childhood. Thus, he begins to translate, and there is set up a new neurophysiological process: *indirect language learning*.

It is not all a matter of age, for second languages are frequently taught by the indirect school method even to children before the age of nine. The teacher whose mother tongue was English, and who must explain French to little children using English to do so, is using the indirect method of teaching. She instructs them, not only because of her method but also by her pronunciation, to speak French with units that belong to the English tongue. She teaches them to learn by the indirect method and to speak by it.

The teacher whose mother tongue was French and who enters the class room and talks only in French, even though she makes no effort to do anything but play with them, allows the children to learn by the direct method and to acquire French speech units that can be used later, should they have the opportunity of expanding French vocabulary. They think in the new language from the beginning.

The indirect method of language teaching has been borrowed by educators from the methods that were developed for the teaching of Latin and Greek. These two languages, once the only link men had with the rich culture of the classical past, gradually ceased to be spoken and so became "dead languages."

Educators have often declared that the mental discipline involved is excellent. I agree with that. The same may be said, of course, in favor of the four-mile walk between home and the little red schoolhouse of yesterday.

Certainly there is a growing place in the educational scheme for the indirect method of teaching secondary languages in high school and university. It would achieve more if direct language learning could be used as an introduction to it. There is also an almost totally ignored opportunity for the use of the direct method of teaching secondary languages at an earlier age level.

My purpose here, it should be stated, at the close of this discussion of the indirect method, is merely to point out the differences in the brain physiology of the two methods. The planning of teaching methods and curricula is the task of the expert educator. If these discussions of the physiology and psychology of language learning have practical value for teaching, he will know best what practical application to make.

2. *Language learning by the direct method.* The mechanism that is developed in the brain is the same whether one, two, or more languages are learned. French is not subserved by one area of brain and English and Chinese by others, in spite of the fact that cases have been published of adults who lost one language and preserved another as the result of "stroke" or other injury to the brain. Our conclusion is that these patients must have been inadequately studied, or else there were psychological reasons why one language was preferred in the recovery period. After thirty years of experience in the bilingual community of Montreal, I have never seen such an example. We have often been told, even by physicians, that this patient or that patient has lost his French but not his English, or vice versa. But careful examination has proven invariably that such judgments were false.

A child who is exposed to two or three languages during the ideal period for language beginning, pronounces each with the accent of his teacher. If he hears one language at home, another at school, and a third, perhaps, with a governess in the nursery, he is not aware that he is learning three languages at all. He is aware of the fact that to get what he wants with the governess he must speak one way, and with his teacher he must speak in another way. He does not reason it out at all. There is no French, no German, no English. It is simpler than that.

Although the cortico-thalamic speech mechanism serves all three languages and there is no evidence of anatomical separation, nevertheless, there is a curiously effective automatic switch that allows each individual to turn from one language to another. What I have referred to as a "switch" would be called, by experimental physiologists, a conditioned reflex. When child or adult turns to an individual who speaks only English, he speaks English, and, turning to a man who speaks French and hearing a word of French, the conditioning signal turns the switch over and only French words come to mind. During multiple language learning it would seem to be best for the learner that his environment should not vary too much. Teachers who teach language should speak only one language.

3. *Language learning by the mother's method.* The best use of

253

the direct method of teaching language is that employed in the home. The method of teaching children their mother's own language has been much the same in all lands and in all ages. It is extraordinarily efficient. It conforms to the changing capacities of the child's brain. The mother's method is the original direct method. It has also been used by servants and tutors in the home to teach one, two, or more secondary languages from the beginning of history. This makes it seem the more surprising that educators today do not generally employ the method in schools.

The mother's method is simple. It is familiar to everyone. Nevertheless, let us examine it. Even before the child understands, the mother talks to him. Before he speaks she watches for understanding. When he says his first words he has a delighted audience. Language is for him only a means to an end, never an end in itself. When he learns about words he is learning about life, learning to get what he wants, learning to share his own exciting ideas with others, learning to understand wonderful fairy tales and exciting facts about trains and trucks and animals and dolls. One secret of the success of this method is, of course, that it is employed while a child is forming the speech units in his eager little brain.

A child who hears three languages instead of one, early enough, learns the units of all three without added effort and without confusion. I have watched this experiment in my own home, as many others must have done.

Our two younger children heard only German in the nursery from the ages of 6 months and 18 months onward because they had a German governess. Even their parents talked German with them, to the best of their ability, when they entered the nursery. At the ages of 3 and 4 they entered a French nursery school. From their parents and others outside the school and outside the nursery they began to hear English gradually.

It was a conditioned reflex for those children, on entering the school room, to utilize the language units of the French tongue; a conditioned reflex on meeting the governess, wherever they found her, to use the German units; from English playmates they learned English. There was no confusion.

After 2 years in the French nursery school they entered a regular English school. In retrospect, it would have been better to continue the French to the age of 7. The seven-year-old "hangs on" to things. In English school too many years elapsed before French and German were presented to them as regular secondary languages. But, nevertheless, they found the work easy and their accents were good. Hidden away in the brain of each were the speech units of all three languages, waiting to be employed in the expansion of a vocabulary which normally takes place in later school-years.

Our two older children heard German first at 8 and 9, when they played with German children for a few months in a small town in Germany. The governess who could speak no English entered the household then. They were never taught German until university level, but in the end they spoke it fluently with a perfect accent.

Of course, there is nothing new in all this. The experiment succeeded. But not all households can include a governess. If public education is to incorporate secondary languages into the curriculum, it should be planned according to the changing aptitudes of the human brain. When new languages are taken up for the first time in the second decade of life, it is difficult, though not impossible, to achieve a good result. It is difficult because it is unphysiological.

G. *Schooling*

In this new day of nationalism and freedom, educators seek, quite rightly, to make education available to all. But unless the mother's method is introduced into the schools, the majority, even of those who are taught, will continue to fail to master any language but their mother tongue.

Bilingualism is not a handicap to a country. It has been a great benefit to mankind, as multilingualism has, also. The language of Greece served the Romans very well as a second language for centuries, and both Greek and Latin were lamps in the great darkness of medieval Europe until the time of the Renaissance. Then, through these two secondary languages, the light of a bygone day flooded the minds of men, who woke, as though from sleep.

The time to begin what might be called a general schooling in secondary languages, in accordance with the demands of brain physiology, is between the ages of 4 and 10. The child sets off for school then, and he can still learn new languages directly without interposing the speech units of his mother tongue.

Suppose we discuss a hypothetical day school in the bilingual community that I know best—that of the city of Montreal and the province of Quebec. A million citizens in Montreal have French for their mother tongue, and less than half that number, English. Suppose the school is located in an English-speaking section of the city. Let the first years, from nursery school and kindergarten on to the grades for children of eight, perhaps, be conducted by teachers whose mother tongue is French.

The French teachers must speak only their native tongue in school, at work, and at organized play, with never a word of translation. Thus the little ones would begin their years of normal play, drawing, singing, and memorizing in French. They would be taught no language as such, but the teachers would "get on" from fairy tales to folk literature as rapidly as the child's mind is prepared for it. These children would have been hearing Mother Goose stories and such things at home, and their play at the weekends, as well as the home discipline and religious observance, would have been carried out in English.

Two or three years of this might well be enough. If so, they could be rotated then into a school or department conducted in another secondary language, if desired.

At the age of 8 or 10 they would graduate, perhaps, into a school conducted in the mother tongue. There they would carry on with all the subjects of a normal curriculum. This would include, in time, courses in the literature of those languages in which their earliest schooling had been presented. They would turn to those subjects effectively and without accent. They would be ready to expand their vocabularies using the language units of understanding and pronunciation learned earlier.

During higher education it will always be desirable that some students take up new languages at a later period, and there is a good deal of evidence that he who has learned more than one language as a little child has greater facility for the acquisition of additional languages in adult life.

There are alternatives to the one I have suggested, of course. One is the language teacher who enters the class for one period every day to speak his or her native tongue. This should begin at age 5 or 6, when children are ready for games and singing if possible.* It would be most effective if there had been at least one pre-liminary year conducted entirely in the second language at kinder-garten level.

Language, when it is learned by the normal physiological process, is not taught at all. It is learned as a by-product of other pursuits. The learner should understand in the language, speak in the language, think in the language, even ignore the language. For the direct learner, language is not a subject to be studied nor an object to be grasped. It is a means to other ends, a vehicle, and a way of life.

My plea to educators and parents is that they should give some thought to the nature of the brain of a child, for the brain is a living mechanism, not a machine. In case of breakdown, it can substitute one of its parts for the function of another. But it has its limitations. It is subject to inexorable change with the passage of time.

In the words of the unknown writer of Ecclesiastes:

"To everything there is a season and a time to every purpose under heaven:

"A time to be born and a time to die. A time to plant and a time to pluck up that which is planted.

.   .   .   .

"A time to weep and a time to laugh; a time to mourn, and a time to dance."

Man's mind has its own peculiar calendar. There is a time to plant, a time to wait on increase, a time for the harvest of knowl-edge, and, at last, a time for wisdom.

* Dr. Robert Gauthier, Director of French Education in the Province of Ontario, has introduced an interesting new method of teaching French to English children in English schools. The method was first described to him by Dr. Tan Gwan Leong, Curriculum Officer of Burma. In Gauthier's experiment the French teacher enters the English class for a period on certain days. He talks in French and the children answer in English, if they choose. This was carried out in fifth and seventh grades, be-ginning with the September opening of the term. At Christmas time half of the children were answering in French. When I visited the experiment, I thought the accent of the children was good, especially in the younger class.

BIBLIOGRAPHY

ℒ. ℛ.

ADRIAN, E. D. 1947. *The Physical Background of Perception.* Oxford, The Clarendon Press, 95 pp.

AJURIAGUERRA, J. DE and HECAEN, H. 1949. *Le Cortex Cerebral; Etude Neuro-psycho-pathologique.* Masson et Cie, Paris, 413 pp.

ALAJOUANINE, T. 1948. Aphasia and artistic realization. *Brain* 71:229-241.

ALAJOUANINE, T., PICHOT, P. and DURAND, M. 1949. Dissociation des altérations phonétiques avec conservation relative de la langue la plus ancient dans un cas d'anarthrie pure chez un sujet français bilingue. *Encéphale* 38:245-265.

ALFORD, L. B. 1948. Cerebral Localization, Outline of a Revision. *Nervous and Mental Disease Monographs. No. 77,* New York, 99 pp.

ALLEN, I. M. 1952. The history of congenital auditory imperception. *N.Z. Med. J.* 51:239-247.

ANDERSON, A. L. 1951. The effect of laterality localization of focal brain lesions on the Wechsler-Bellevue subtests. *J. Clin. Psychol.* 7:149-153.

ARDIN-DELTEIL, LEVI-VALENSI, DERRIEU. 1923. Deux Cas d'Aphasie; I. Aphasie de Broca par lésion de l'hemisphère droit chez une droitière. II. Aphasie avec hémiplégie droite chez une gauchère. *Rev. Neurol.* 1:14-24.

AUSTREGESILO, A. 1940. Aphasie et lobe pariétal gauche. *Pr. Méd.* 48:126-132.

BAILEY, P. 1924. A contribution to the study of aphasia and apraxia. *Arch. Neurol. Psychiat.,* Chicago. 11:501-529.

BALL, A. B. 1881. A contribution to the study of aphasia with special reference to "word-deafness" and "word-blindness." *Arch. Med.* 5:1-26.

BARLOW, T. 1877. On a case of double hemiplegia, with cerebral symmetrical lesions. *Brit. Med. J.* July 28, pp. 103-104.

BARRETT, A. M. 1910. A case of pure word-deafness with autopsy. *J. Nerv. Ment. Dis.* 37:73-92.

BASTIAN, H. C. 1882. *The Brain as an Organ of Mind.* Ed. 3, London, Kegan Paul, Trench & Co., 690 pp.

BASTIAN, H. C. 1897. The Lumelian Lectures on some problems in connection with aphasia and other speech defects. Reprinted from the *Lancet,* April 3, 10, 24 and May 1.

BASTIAN, H. C. 1898. *Aphasia and other Speech Defects.* London, H. K. Lewis, 366 pp.

BATEMAN, F. 1869. On aphasia and the localisation of the faculty of speech. *Med. Times and Gaz.,* pp. 486-488; 540-542.

BATEMAN, F. 1870. *On Aphasia or Loss of Speech and the Localisation of the Faculty of Articulate Language.* London, John Churchill and Sons, 180 pp.

BATTERSBY, W. S., KRIEGER, H. P., POLLACK, M. and BENDER, M. B. 1953. Figure-ground discrimination and the "abstract attitude" in patients with cerebral neoplasms. *Arch. Neurol. Psychiat.*, Chicago. 70:703-712.

BAY, E. 1950. Agnosie und Funktionswandel: Eine Hirnpathologische Studie. Berlin, Springer, *Monogr. Neurol. Psychiat. No. 73*, 194 pp.

BAY, E. 1951. Über den Begriff der Agnosie. *Nervenarzt.* 22:179-187.

BAY, E. 1952. Der gegenwärtige Stand der Aphasieforschung. *Folia Phoniatr.*, Basel. 4:9-29.

BAY, E. 1953. Disturbances of visual perception and their examination. *Brain* 76:515-550.

BAZETT, H. C., and PENFIELD, W. 1922. A study of the Sherrington decerebrate animal in the chronic as well as the acute condition. *Brain* 45:185-264.

BELL, J. 1895. Aphasia with left hemiplegia. *Montreal Med. J.* 24:269.

BERNARD, D. 1885. *De l'Aphasie et de ses Diverses Formes.* Thesis. Paris, V. Goupy et Jourdan, 270 pp.

BERNHEIM, F. 1885. Contribution à l'étude de l'aphasie. De la cécité psychique des choses. *Rev. Méd.*, Paris. 15:625-637.

BERNHEIM, F. 1900. *De l'Aphasie Motrice.* Thesis. Paris, G. Carré et C. Naud, 374 pp.

BERTRAND, G. 1956. Spinal efferent pathways from the supplementary motor area. *Brain* 79:461-473.

BIANCHI, L. 1910. La syndrome pariétale. *Ann. Nevrol.* 28:137-177.

BITOT 1884. Du siège et de la direction des irradiations capsulaires chargées de transmettre la parole. *Arch. Neurol.*, Paris. 8:1-22; 151-173.

BLAU, A. 1946. The Master Hand. *Research Monographs, No. 5.* American Orthopsychiatric Association, New York. Amer. Orthopsychiat. Assoc. Inc., 206 pp.

BOUILLAUD, J. 1825. Recherches cliniques propres à démontrer que la perte de la parole correspond à la lesion des lobules antérieurs du cerveau, et à confirmer l'opinion de M. Gall, sur le siège de l'organs du langage articulé. *Arch. Gén. Méd.* 8:25-45.

BOUILLAUD, J. 1865. Discussion sur la faculté du langage articulé. *Bull. Acad. Méd.*, Paris. 30:575-600; 604-638.

BRAIN, W. R. 1941a. Visual object-agnosia with special reference to the Gestalt theory. *Brain* 64:43-62.

BRAIN, W. R. 1941b. Visual disorientation with special reference to lesions of the right cerebral hemisphere. *Brain* 64:244-272.

BRAIN, W. R. 1945. Speech and handedness. *Lancet* 2:837-841.

BRAIN, W. R. 1955. Aphasia, Apraxia and Agnosia. In Wilson, K. *Neurology.* London, Butterworth, Vol. III, pp. 1413-1483.

BRAMWELL, B. 1898. A remarkable case of aphasia. *Brain* 21:343-373.

BRAMWELL, B. 1899. On "crossed" aphasia and the factors which go to determine whether the "leading" or "driving" speech-centres shall be located in the left or in the right hemisphere of the brain. With notes on a case of "crossed" aphasia (aphasia with right-sided hemiplegia) in a left-handed man. *Lancet* 1:1473-1479.

BRAMWELL, E. 1927. A case of cortical deafness. *Brain* 50:579-580.

BRICKNER, R. M. 1940. A human cortical area producing repetitive phenomena when stimulated. *J. Neurophysiol.* 3:128-130.

BROADBENT, W. H. 1872. On the cerebral mechanism of speech and thought. *Med.-Chi. Trans.* 15:145-194.

BROADBENT, W. H. 1878. A case of peculiar affection of speech, with commentary. *Brain* 1:484-503.

BROCA, P. 1888. *Mémoires sur le Cerveau de l'Homme.* With introduction by S. Pozzi. Paris, C. Reinwald, pp. 1-161.

BROWN, T. GRAHAM and SHERRINGTON, C. S. 1912. On the instability of a cortical point. *Proc. Roy. Soc.*, B. 85:250-277.

BROWN-SÉQUARD, C. E. 1877. Aphasia as an effect of brain-disease. *Dublin J. Med. Sci.* March, pp. 1-18.

BRUCE, W. 1868. Case of partial aphasia with left hemiplegia. *Med. Times and Gaz.* I:87-88.

BUCY, P. C. 1951. Discussion of paper by Erickson and Woolsey (1951). *Trans. Amer. Neurol. Assoc.*, p. 57.

BUCY, P. C. and CASE, T. J. 1937. Athetosis II. Surgical treatment of unilateral athetosis. *Arch. Neurol. Psychiat.*, Chicago. 37:983-1020.

BURCKHARDT, G. 1891. Ueber Rindenexcisionen, als Beitrag zur operativen Therapie der Psychosen. *Allg. Z. Psychiat.* 47:463-548.

CAIRNS, H., OLDFIELD, R. C., PENNYBACKER, F. B. and WHITTERIDGE, D. 1941. Akinetic mutism with an epidermoid cyst of the 3rd ventricle. *Brain* 64:273-290.

CAMPBELL, A. W. 1905. *Histological Studies on the Localisation of Cerebral Function.* Cambridge University Press, 360 pp.

CAMPION, G. G. and SMITH, G. E. 1934. *The Neural Basis of Thought.* London, Kegan Paul and Trench, 151 pp.

CHARCOT, J. P. 1883. Des différentes formes de l'aphasie — de la cécité verbale. *Progr. Méd.*, Paris. 11:441-444.

CHARCOT, J. P. 1883. Des varietés de l'aphasie. I. De la cécité des mots. II. Aphasie motrice. *Progr. Méd.*, Paris. 11:469-471; 487-488; 521-523; 859-861.

CHARCOT, J. P. 1890. *Oeuvres Complètes de J. M. Charcot.* Paris, Lecrosnier et Babé, Vol. 3, pp. 154-192.

CHAVANY, J-A. 1945. Un cas de surdité d'origine corticale. *Progr. Méd.*, Paris. 53:472.

CHESHER, E. C. 1936. Some observations concerning the relation of handedness to the language mechanism. *Bull. Neurol. Inst. N.Y.* 4:556-562.

CHESHER, E. C. 1937. Aphasia I. Technique of clinical examinations. *Bull. Neurol. Inst. N.Y.* 6:134-144.

CLARK, W. E. LeGROS and RUSSELL, W. R. 1938. Cortical deafness without aphasia. *Brain* 61:375-383.

CHUSID, J. G., GUTIÉRREZ-MAHONEY, C. G. de and MARGULES-LAVERGNE, M. P. 1954. Speech disturbances in association with parasagittal frontal lesions. *J. Neurosurg.* 11:193-204.

CLAUDE, H. and SCHAEFFER, H. 1921. Un nouveau cas d'hémiplégie gauche avec aphasie chez un droitier. *Rev. Neurol.* 28:170-175.

COBB, S. 1943. *Borderlines of Psychiatry.* Cambridge, Mass., Harvard University Press, 166 pp.

COBB, S. 1944. *Fundamentals of Neuropsychiatry.* Ed. 3. Baltimore, William Wood, 252 pp.

COLUMELLA, F. and PAPO, I. 1953. Contributo allo studio della aprassia construttiva. *Arch. Psicol. Neur. Psich.* 14:390-403.

CONRAD, K. 1949. Über aphasische Sprachstörungen bei hirnverletzten Linkshändern. *Nervenarzt* 20:148-154.

CONRAD, K. 1951. Aphasie, Agnosie, Apraxie. *Fortschr. Neur. Psychiat.* 19:291-325.

CRITCHLEY, M. 1930. The anterior cerebral artery, and its syndromes. *Brain* 53:120-165.

CRITCHLEY, M. 1938. "Aphasia" in a partial deaf-mute. *Brain* 61:163-169.

CRITCHLEY, M. 1942. Aphasic disorders of signalling (constitutional and acquired) occurring in naval signalmen. *J. Mt. Sinai Hosp.* 9:363-375.

CRITCHLEY, M. 1953. *The Parietal Lobes.* London, Edward Arnold & Co., 480 pp.

CRITCHLEY, M. 1954. Parietal syndromes in ambidextrous and left-handed subjects. *Zbl. Neurochir.* 14:4-16.

CROSS, T. M. B. 1872. Amnesic and ataxic aphasia with agraphia and temporary right hemiplegia, the result of embolism of the left middle cerebral artery. *Amer. Practit.*, April, pp. 1-13.

CUFFER 1880. Hémiplégie gauche avec aphasie chez une femme gauchère et récemment accouchée—Troubles de la sécrétion lactée; suppression de cette sécrétion dans le sein droit, exagération de la sécrétion lactée dans le sein gauche. *France Méd.* 27:217-218.

CUMMINS, H. 1940. Finger prints correlated with handedness. *Amer. J. Phys. Anthrop.* 26:151-166.

CUSHING, H. 1909. A note upon the faradic stimulation of the post-central gyrus in conscious patients. *Brain* 32:44-53.

CUSHING, H. and EISENHARDT, L. 1938. *Meningiomas:Their Classification, Regional Behaviour, Life History, and Surgical End Results.* Springfield, Ill., Charles C. Thomas, 785 pp.

DALLY 1882. Observation d'aphasie avec hémiplégie gauche. *Ann. Méd.-Psychol.*, Paris 8:252-253.

DATTNER, B., DAVIS, V. T. and SMITH, C. E. 1952. A case of subcortical visual verbal agnosia. *J. Nerv. Ment. Dis.* 116:808-811.

DAX, M. 1865. Lésions de la moitié gauche de l'encéphale coincident avec l'oubli des signes de la pensée. Montpellier, 1836. *Gaz. Hebdom*, 1865. S2, 11:259-260.

DEJERINE, J. 1892. Contribution à l'étude anatomo-pathologique et clinique des différentes varietés de cécité verbale. *Mém. Soc. Biol.* Fév.27. Abstract in *Brain* 16:318-320, 1893.

DEJERINE, Madame J. 1908. Discussion sur l'aphasie, Société de Neurologie de Paris. *Rev. Neurol.* 16:974-1024.

DEJERINE, J. 1914. *Sémiologie des Affections du Système Nerveux*. Paris, Masson et Cie. pp. 68-166.

DEJERINE, J. and ANDRE-THOMAS 1912. Contribution à l'étude de l'aphasie chez les gauchers et des dégénérations du corps calleux. *Rev. Neurol.* 24:313-326.

DENNY-BROWN, D. 1951. The frontal lobes and their functions. In *Modern Trends in Neurology*, edited by Feiling, A., London, Butterworth and Co., pp. 13-89.

DENNY-BROWN, D. and BANKER, B. Q. 1954. Amorphosynthesis from left parietal lesion. *Arch. Neurol. Psychiat.*, Chicago. 71:302-313.

DENNY-BROWN, D., MEYER, J. S. and HORENSTEIN, S. 1952. The significance of perceptual rivalry resulting from parietal lesion. *Brain* 75:433-471.

DIMITRI, V. 1933. *Afasias Estudio Anátomoclínico*. Buenos Aires, El Ateneo, 188 pp.

Discussion sur la faculté du langage articulé. 1865. *Bull. Acad. Méd.*, Paris. 30:679-703.

Discussion sur l'aphasie. Sociéte de Neurologie de Paris. 1908. *Rev. Neurol.* 16:611-636; 974-1074.

DUENSING, F. 1953. I. Zur Frage der Buchstabenalexie. II. Über die Wortalexie. III. Über Alexie mit partiell erhaltenem simultanen Wortlesen. *Arch. Psychiat. Nervenkr.* 191:147-190.

ECCLES, J. 1951. Hypotheses relating to the brain-mind problem. *Nature* 168:53-65.

ELDER, W. 1897. *Aphasia and the Cerebral Speech Mechanism*. London, H. K. Lewis, 259 pp.

ELSBERG, C. A. 1931. The parasagittal meningeal fibroblastomas. *Bull. Neurol. Inst., N.Y.* 1:389-418.

ELVIN, M. B. and OLDFIELD, R. C. 1951. Disabilities and progress in a dysphasic university student. *J. Neurol. Psychiat.* 14:118-128.

ERICKSON, T. C. and WOOLSEY, C. N. 1951. Observations on the supplementary motor area of man. *Trans. Amer. Neurol. Assoc.* 76:50-56.

ETHELBERG, S. 1951. On changes in circulation through the anterior cerebral artery. A clinical-angiographical study. *Acta Psychiat.*, Supp. 75, 211 pp.

ETTLINGER, G., JACKSON, C. V. and ZANGWILL, O. L. 1955. Dysphasia following right temporal lobectomy in a right-handed man. *J. Neurol. Psychiat.* 18:214-217.

ETTLINGER, G., JACKSON, C. V. and ZANGWILL, O. L. 1956. Cerebral dominance in sinistrals. *Brain* 79:569-588.

EUSTIS, R. S. 1949. Right- or left-handedness. A practical problem. *New Engl. J. Med.* 240:249-253.

FEINDEL, W. and PENFIELD, W. 1954. Localization of discharge in temporal lobe automatism. *Arch. Neurol. Psychiat.,* Chicago. 72:605-630.

FERRIER, D. 1886. *The Functions of the Brain.* Ed. 2. London, Smith, Elder & Co. 498 pp.

FESSARD, A. E. 1954. Mechanisms of nervous integration and conscious experience. In *Brain Mechanisms and Consciousness.* Edited by Adrian and others. Oxford, Blackwell Scientific Publications. pp. 200-237.

FINKELNBURG, F. C. 1870. Niederrheinische Gesellschaft, Sitzung vom 21 März, 1870 in Bonn. *Berlin Klin. Wochenschr.* 449-450; 460-462. Cited by Kussmaul (1877).

FISHER, R. A. 1950. *Statistical Method for Research Workers.* New York, Hafner Pub. Co., 354 pp.

FLOURENS, P. 1824. *Recherches Expérimentales sur les Propriétés et les Fonctions du Système Nerveux dans les Animaux Vertébrés.* Paris, Crevot, 332 pp.

FOERSTER, O. 1936. Motorische Felder und Bahnen. In Bumke und Foerster: *Handbuch der Neurologie.* Berlin, Julius Springer, 6:1-357.

FOERSTER, O. and PENFIELD, W. 1930a. The structural basis of traumatic epilepsy and results of radical operation. *Brain* 53:99-120.

FOERSTER, O. and PENFIELD, W. 1930b. Der Narbenzug am und im Gehirn bei traumatischer Epilepsie in seiner Bedeutung für das Zustandekommen der Anfälle und für die therapeutische Bekampfung derselben. *Z. ges. Neurol. Psychiat.* 125:475-572.

FOULIS, D. 1879. A case in which there was destruction of the third left frontal convolution without aphasia. *Brit. Med. J.* 1:383.

FOX, J. C., Jr. and GERMAN, W. J. 1935. Observations following left (dominant) temporal lobectomy. *Arch. Neurol. Psychiat.,* Chicago. 33:791-806.

FREUD, S. 1891. *Zur Auffassung der Aphasien.* Leipzig and Vienna, Franz Deuticke, 107 pp. Translated by E. Stengel. *On Aphasia, a critical study.* New York, International University Press, 105 pp.

FREUND, C. S. 1888. Über optische Aphasie und Seelenblindheit. *Arch. Psychiat. Nervenkr.* 20:276-297.

FRIEDMAN, E. D. 1934. Neurological aspects of hoarseness. *N.Y. St. J. Med.* 34:48-50.

FRITSCH, G. and HITZIG, E. 1870. Ueber die elektrische Erregbarkeit des Grosshirns. *Arch. Anat. Physiol.,* Lpz. 37:300-332.

GALL, F. J. and SPURZHEIM, G. 1810-1819. *Anatomie et Physiologie du Système Nerveux en Général et du Cerveau en Particulier.* Paris, Schoell, 320 pp.

GARDNER, W. J. 1941. Injection of procaine into the brain to locate speech area in left-handed persons. *Arch. Neurol. Psychiat.*, Chicago. 46:1035-1038.

GASTAUT, H. 1955. Physiopathogénie des épilepsies. *Assemblée Française de Médecine Générale.* 13:259-262.

GELLER, W. 1952. Über Lokalisationsfragen bei Rechenstörungen. *Fortschr. Neur. Psychiat.* 20:173-194.

GERMAN, W. J. and Fox, J. C., Jr. 1934. Observations following unilateral lobectomies. *Res. Publ. Assoc. Nerv. Ment. Dis.* 13:378-434.

GERSTMANN, J. 1927. Fingeragnosie und isolierte Agraphie—ein neues Syndrom. *Z. Neurol. Psychiat.* 108:152-177.

GESELL, A. and ILG, F. L. 1946. *The Child from Five to Ten.* New York, Harpers, pp. 444-449.

GLOOR, P. 1955. Electrophysiological studies on the connections of the amygdaloid nucleus in the cat. Part II. Electrophysiological properties of amygdaloid projection system. *Electroenceph. Clin. Neurophysiol.* 7:243-264.

GOLDSTEIN, K. 1948. *Language and Language Disturbances.* New York, Grune and Stratton, 374 pp.

GOLDSTEIN, K. and GELB, A. 1918. Psychologische Analysen hirnpathologischer Fälle auf Grund von Untersuchungen Hirnverletzter. I. Abhandlung zur Psychologie des optischen Wahrnehmungs—und Erkennungs—vorganges. *Z. ges. Neurol. Psychiat.* 41:1-142.

GOODDY, W. and McKISSOCK, W. 1951. The theory of cerebral localisation. *Lancet* 1:481-483.

GOODGLASS, H. and QUADFASEL, F. A. 1954. Language laterality in left-handed patients. *Brain* 77:521-548.

GORDINIER, H. C. 1899. A case of brain tumor at the base of the second left frontal convolution. *Amer. J. Med. Sci.* 117:526-535.

GORDINIER, H. C. 1903. Arguments in favour of the existence of a separate center for writing. *Amer. J. Med. Sci.* 126:490-503.

GOWERS, W. R. 1893. *A Manual of Diseases of the Nervous System.* Ed. 2. London, J. and A. Churchill, Vol. 2, pp. 109-125.

GUIDETTI, B. 1957. Désordres de la parole associés à des lésions de la surface interhémisphèrique frontale postérieure. *Rev. Neurol.* 97:121-131.

GUTTMAN, E. 1942. Aphasia in children. *Brain* 65:205-219.

HABERSHON, 1880. A case of aphasia with hemiplegia on the left side and tumour on the right side of the brain in the third frontal convolution. *Brit. Med. J.* II:1015-1016; and the same case, *Med. Times & Gaz.* 21, 1881.

HAMMOND, W. A. 1871. On aphasia. *Med. Rec.*, New York. March, pp. 1-6 and p. 19.

HARTMANN, A. 1889. Beitrag zur Lehre von der Aphasie. *Med. Klinik zu Kiel* 5:5-28.

HEAD, H. 1915. Hughlings Jackson on aphasia and kindred affections of speech. *Brain* 38:1-27.

HEAD, H. 1926. *Aphasia and Kindred Disorders of Speech*. London, Cambridge University Press, 2 vols.

HEBB, D. O. 1939. Intelligence in man after large removals of cerebral tissue: Report of four left frontal lobe cases. *J. Genet. Psychol.* 21:73-87.

HEBB, D. O. 1942a. The effect of early and late brain injury upon test scores, and the nature of normal adult intelligence. *Proc. Amer. Phil. Soc.* 85:275-292.

HEBB, D. O. 1942b. Verbal test material independent of special vocabulary difficulty. *J. Educ. Psychol.* 33:691-696.

HEBB, D. O. 1949. *The Organization of Behavior*. New York, John Wiley and Sons, Inc., 319 pp.

HEBB, D. O. and MORTON, N. W. 1943. The McGill adult comprehension examination: "Verbal situation" and "picture anomaly" series. *J. Educ. Psychol.* 34:16-25.

HEBB, D. O. and PENFIELD, W. 1940. Human behavior after extensive bilateral removal from the frontal lobes. *Arch. Neurol. Psychiat.*, Chicago. 44:421-438.

HECAEN, H., AJURIAGUERRA, J. de, MAGIS, C. and ANGELERGUES, R. 1952. Le problème de l'agnosie des physionomies. *Encéphale* 41:322-355.

HECAEN, H., PENFIELD, W., BERTRAND, C. and MALMO, R. 1956. The syndrome of apractognosia due to lesions of the minor cerebral hemisphere. *Arch. Neurol. Psychiat.*, Chicago. 75:400-434.

HEILLY, E. and CHANTEMESSE, A. 1883. Note sur un cas de cécité et de surdité verbales. *Progr. Méd.*, Paris. 11:22-25.

HEINE 1903. Amnestische Aphasie und Hemiopie in Folge von Abszess des rechten Schläfen und Hinterhauptlappens. *Deutsch Med. Wschr.*, p. 221.

HEMPHILL, R. E. and STENGEL, E. 1940. A study of pure word-deafness. *J. Neurol. Psychiat.* 3:251-262.

HENSCHEN, S. E. 1918. Über die Hörsphäse. *J. Psychol. Neurol.*, Lpz. 22:319-474.

HENSCHEN, S. E. 1920-1922. *Klinische und Anatomische Beitrage zur Pathologie des Gehirns*. Stockholm, Nordiska Bokhandeln, Vol. 5, Vol. 6, Henschen, Vol. 7.

HENSCHEN, S. E. 1925. Clinical and anatomical contributions on brain pathology. Abstracts and comments by W. F. Schaller. *Arch. Neurol. Psychiat.*, Chicago. 13:226-249.

HENSCHEN, S. E. 1926. On the function of the right hemisphere of the brain in relation to the left in speech, music and calculation. *Brain* 49:110-123.

HERRMANN, G. and PÖTZL, O. 1926. *Über die Agraphie und ihre lokal-diagnostischen Beziehungen.* Berlin, Karger, 380 pp.

HERRICK, C. J. 1955. Psychology from a biologist's point of view. *Psychol. Rev.* 62:333-340.

HERVEY, R. 1874. Maladie de Bright—Dsypnée urémique.—Apoplexie pulmonaire.—Aphasie, hémiplégie faciale droite.—Hydropneumo-thorax.—Mort.—Lésion limitée à la 3e circonvolution frontale gauche. *Bull. Soc. Anat.*, Paris. 49:29-34.

HEUBNER, O. 1899. Aphasie. *Schmidt's Jahrbüch ges. Med.* 224:220-222.

HEUYER, G. and FELD, M. 1954. Hémisphèrectomie gauche pour atrophie cicatricielle chez un enfant droitier. Discussion de l'acquisition postopératoire du langage. *Rev. Neurol.* 90:52-58.

HILLIER, W. F., Jr. 1954. Total left cerebral hemispherectomy for malignant glioma. *Neurology* 4:718-721.

HOLMES, G. 1918. Disturbances of vision by cerebral lesions. *Brit. J. Ophthal.* 2:353-383.

HOLMES, G. 1919. Lecture II. Disturbance of visual space perception. *Brit. Med. J.* 2:230-233.

HOLMES, G. 1950. Pure word blindness. *Folia Psychiat.* 53:279-288.

HOLMES, G. and HORRAX, G. 1919. Disturbances of spatial orientation and visual attention, with loss of stereoscopic vision. *Arch. Neurol. Psychiat.*, Chicago. 1:385-407.

Holy Bible, King James version, Judges 20:16.

HORDIJK, W. 1952. Epilepsie en links-handigheid. *Ned. Tijdschr. Geneesk.* 96:263-269.

HUMPHREY, M. E. and ZANGWILL, O. L. 1952a. Dysphasia in left-handed patients with unilateral brain lesions. *J. Neurol. Psychiat.* 15:184-193.

HUMPHREY, M. E. and ZANGWILL, O. L. 1952b. Effects of a right-sided occipito-parietal brain injury in a left-handed man. *Brain* 75:312-324.

HUTTER, K. 1951. Auswirkung der Händigkeit bei erbgleichen Zwillingen. *Med. Klin.* 46:503-504.

HYLAND, H. H. 1933. Thrombosis of intracranial arteries. Report of those cases involving, respectively, the anterior cerebral, basilar and internal carotid arteries. *Arch. Neurol. Psychiat.*, Chicago. 30:342-356.

INGHAM, S. D. and NIELSEN, J. M. 1937. Interpretation dissociated from recognition of visual symbols; illustrated by case of complete major (left) temporal lobectomy. *Bull. Los Angeles Neurol. Soc.* 2:1-10.

JACKSON, J. Hughlings 1864. Loss of speech; its association with valvular disease of the heart and with hemiplegia on the right side. *Lond. Hosp. Rep.* 1:388-471.

JACKSON, J. Hughlings 1868. Defect of intellectual expression (aphasia) with left hemiplegia. *Lancet* 1:457.

JACKSON, J. Hughlings 1880. On aphasia, with left hemiplegia. *Lancet* 1:637-638.

JACKSON, J. Hughlings 1890. Lumelian Lectures on convulsive seizures. *Brit. Med. J.* 1:412.

JACKSON, J. Hughlings 1915. Hughlings Jackson on aphasia and kindred affections of speech, together with a complete bibliography of his publications on speech and a reprint of some of the more important papers. *Brain* 38:1-190.

JACKSON, J. Hughlings 1931. *Selected Writings of John Hughlings Jackson.* Edited by James Taylor. London, Hodder and Stoughton. Vol. 2, pp. 121-212.

JAMES, W. 1910. *The Principles of Psychology.* New York. Henry Holt and Co.

JASPER, H. H. and PENFIELD, W. 1949. Electrocorticograms in man: Effect of voluntary movement upon the electrical activity of the precentral gyrus. *Arch. Psychiat. Nervenkr.* 183:163-174.

JEFFERSON, G. 1935. Jacksonian epilepsy. A background and a postscript. *Post-Grad. Med. J.*, London. 11:150-162.

JEFFERSON, G. 1950. Localization of function in the cerebral cortex. *Brit. Med. Bull.* 6:333-340.

JELGERSMA, G. *Atlas anatomicum cerebri humani.* Scheltema and Holkema, Amsterdam.

KARLIN, I. W. 1954. Aphasias in children. *Amer. J. Dis. Child.* 87:752-767.

KENNEDY, F. 1911. The symptomatology of temporosphenoidal tumors. *Arch. Intern. Med.* 8:317-350.

KENNEDY, F. 1916. Stock-brainedness, the causative factor in the so-called "crossed aphasias." *Amer. J. Med. Sci.* 152:849-859.

KENNEDY, F. and WOLF, A. 1936. Relationship of intellect to speech defects in aphasic patients, with illustrative cases. *J. Nerv. Ment. Dis.* 84:125-145; 293-311.

KENNEDY, L. 1947. Remedial procedures for handling aphasic patients. *Arch. Neurol. Psychiat.*, Chicago. 57:646-649.

KLEIN, R. 1937. Über ein parietales Störungssyndrom. *Z. ges. Neurol. Psychiat.* 160:417-425.

KLEIN, R. and STACK, J. J. 1953. Visual agnosia and alternating dominance, analysis of a case. *J. Ment. Sci.* 99:749-762.

KLEIST, K. 1934. *Gehirnpathologie.* Leipzig, Johann Ambrosius Barth, pp. 623-934.

KNJAIZINSKIJ 1927. Cited by Ludwig, C. 1938.

KRYNAUW, R. A. 1950. Infantile hemiplegia treated by removing one cerebral hemisphere. *J. Neurol. Psychiat.* 13:243-267.

KÖSTER, H. 1889-1890. Aphasie bei einem Linkshänder mit wortblindheit. Läsion der rechten Gehirnhemisphäre. *Uppsala LäkForen. Förh.* 5:128-129.

KUBIC, C. S. and ADAMS, R. D. 1946. Occlusion of the basilar artery. A clinical and pathological study. *Brain* 69:73-121.

KÜENBURG, M. von 1930. Zuordnungsversuche bei Gesunden und Sprachgestörten. *Arch. ges. Psychol.* 76:257-352.

KUSSMAUL, A. 1877. Disturbances of Speech. In *Cyclopaedia of the Practice of Medicine*. Edited by H. von Ziemssen, translated by J. A. McCreery, New York, William Wood and Company. 14:581-875.

LASHLEY, K. S. 1948. The mechanism of vision: XVIII. Effects of destroying the visual "associative areas" of the monkey. *Genet. Psychol. Monogr.* 37:107-166.

LASHLEY, K. S. 1952. Functional interpretation of anatomic patterns. *Res. Publ. Assoc. Nerv. & Ment. Dis.* 30:529-547.

LEISCHNER, A. 1943. Die "Aphasie" der Taubstummen. Ein Beitrag zur Lehre von der Asymbolie. *Arch. Psychiat. Nervenkr.* 115:469-548.

LELUT, 1864. Rapport sur le mémoire de M. Dax, relatif aux fonctions de l'hémisphère gauche du cerveau. *Bull. Acad. Méd.* 30:173-175.

LEOPOLD, W. F. 1939-1949. *Speech Development of a Bilingual Child*. Evanston, Ill. Northwestern Univ. Press, 4 vols.

LEWANDOWSKY 1911. Rechtshirnigkeit bei einem Rechtshänder. *Z. ges. Neurol. Psychiat.* 4:1046-1047.

LEYTON, A. S. F. and SHERRINGTON, C. S. 1917. Observations on the excitable cortex of the chimpanzee, orangutan, and gorilla. *Quart. J. Exp. Physiol.* 11:135-222.

LHERMITE, J. 1937. *Les Méchanismes du Cerveau*. Paris, Gallimard, 234 pp.

LICHTHEIM, L. 1885. On aphasia. *Brain* 7:433-484.

LIEPMANN, H. 1912. Anatomische Befunde bei Aphasischen und Apraktischen. *Neurol. Zbl.* 31:1524-1530.

LIEPMANN, H. and MAAS, O. 1907. Fall von linksseitige Agraphie und Apraxie bei rechtsseitiger Lähmung. *J. Psychol. Neurol.*, Lpz. 10:214-227.

LISSAUER, H. 1890. Ein Fall von Seelenblindheit nebst einem Beitrage zur Théorie derselben. *Arch. Psychiat. Nervenkr.* 21:222-270.

LONG, E. 1913. Aphasie par lesion de l'hémisphère gauche chez un gaucher. *Rev. Neurol.* 25:339.

LORDAT, J. 1843-1844. Analyse de la parole pour servir à la théorie de divers cas d'alalie et de paralalie. *J. Soc. Pr.*, Montpellier 7 and 8. Paris, Baillière.

LOVELL, H. W., WAGGONER, R. W. and KAHN, E. A. 1932. Critical study of a case of aphasia. *Arch. Neurol. Psychiat.*, Chicago. 28:1178-1181.

LUDWIG, E. and KLINGLER, J. 1956. *Atlas Cerebri Humani*. Basel, S. Karger, 137 pp.

LUDWIG, M. E. 1938. Beitrag zur Frage der Bedeutung der unterwertigen Hemisphäre. *Z. ges. Neurol. Psychiat.* 164:735-747.

LYMAN, R. S., KWAN, S. T. and CHAO, W. H. 1938. Left occipito-parietal brain tumor with observations on alexia and agraphia, in Chinese and English. *Chin. Med. J.* 54:491-516.

McFIE, J. 1952. Cerebral dominance in cases of reading disability. *J. Neurol. Psychiat.* 15:194-199.

McFIE, J. and PIERCY, M. F. 1952. The relation of laterality of lesion to performance on Weigl's sorting test. *J. Ment. Sci.* 98:299-305.

McFIE, J., PIERCY, M. F. and ZANGWILL, O. L. 1950. Visual spatial agnosia associated with lesions of the right cerebral hemisphere. *Brain* 73:167-190.

MAGNAN 1879-1880. On simple aphasia, and aphasia with incoherence. *Brain* 2:112-123.

MAHOUDEAU, D., DAVIS, M. and LECOEUR, J. 1951. Un nouveau cas d'agraphie sans aphasie, révélatrice d'une tumeur métastique du pied de la deuzième circonvolution frontale gauche. *Rev. Neurol.* 84:159-161.

MARIE, P. 1906. La troisième circumconvolution frontale gauche ne joue aucun rôle spécial dans la fonction du langage. *Sem. Médicale* 26:241-247.

MARIE, P. 1926. *Travaux et Mémoires.* Paris, Masson et Cie., pp. 1-181.

MARIE, P., BOUTTIER, H. and BAILEY, P. 1922a. La Plantotopokinésie. *Rev. Neurol.* 38:505-512.

MARIE, P., BOUTTIER, H. and BAILEY, P. 1922b. Apropos des faits décrits sous le nom d'apraxie ideomotrice. *Rev. Neurol.* 38:973-985.

MARIE, P. and FOIX, C. 1917. Les aphasies de guerre. *Rev. Neurol.* 1:53-87.

MARINESCU, G., GRIGORESCU, D. and AXENTE, S. 1938. Considérations sur l'aphasie croisée. *Encéphale* 33:27-46.

MESNET 1882. Discussion on aphasia in Société Médico-psychologique, 22 May, 1882. *Ann. Méd.-psychol.*, Paris, 8:253.

METTLER, F. A. 1949. *Selective Partial Ablation of the Frontal Cortex: A Correlative Study of the Effects on Human Psychotic Subjects.* New York, Paul B. Hoeber, Inc., 502 pp.

MEYER, S. 1908. Apraktische Agraphie bei einem Rechtshirner. *Zbl. Nervenheilk.* pp. 673-678.

MEYER, V. and YATES, A. J. 1955. Intellectual changes following temporal lobectomy for psychomotor epilepsy. Preliminary communication. *J. Neurol. Psychiat.* 18:44-52.

MEYER, W. 1909. Volständige sensorische Aphasie bei Läsion der rechten ersten Schläfenwindung. *Deut. Med. Wschr.* II:1262-1263.

MEYERS, R. 1948. Relation of "thinking" and language. *Arch. Neurol. Psychiat.*, Chicago, 60:119-139.

MILLER, H. 1950. Discussion on speech defects in children. *Proc. Roy. Soc. Med.* 43:579-582.

MILLS, C. K. 1891. Aphasia and other affections of speech, in some of their medico-legal relations, studied largely from the standpoint of localization. *Rev. Insan. and Nerv. Dis.*, September and December, pp. 1-81.

MILLS, C. K. 1891. On the localisation of the auditory centre. *Brain* 14:465-472.

MILLS, C. K. 1895. The Anatomy of the Cerebral Cortex and the Localization of its Functions. In Dercum, F. X.: *A Textbook on Nervous Diseases* by American Authors. Philadelphia, Lea Brothers and Co., pp. 381-443.

MILLS, C. K. and WEISENBURG, T. H. 1905. Word-blindness, with the record of a case due to a lesion in the right cerebral hemisphere in a right-handed man; with some discussion of the treatment of visual aphasia. *Medicine* 2:822-828.

MILNER, B. 1954. Intellectual function of the temporal lobes. *Psychol. Bull.* 51:42-62.

MILNER, B. and PENFIELD, W. 1955. The effect of hippocampal lesions on recent memory. *Trans. Amer. Neurol. Assoc.* pp. 42-48.

MINKOWSKI, M. 1928. Sur un cas d'aphasie chez un polyglotte. *Rev. Neurol.* 1:362-366.

MISCH, W. 1928. Über corticale Taubheit. *Z. ges. Neurol. Psychiat.* 115:567-573.

MIYAKE, H. 1909. Ein Fall von traumatischer Aphasie mit rechtsseitiger Hemiplegie bei Linkshändigen. Trepanation. Heilung. *Arch. Klin. Chir.* 88:800-810.

MONOKOW, C. von 1897. Gehirnpathologie. In Nothnagel, H.: *Spezielle Pathologie und Therapie*. Vienna, Alfred Hölder. Band IX, Teil I, pp. 482-579.

MONAKOW, C. von 1914. *Die Lokalisation im Grosshirn und der Abbau der Funktion durch corticale Herde*. Wiesbaden, J. F. Bergmann, 1033 pp.

MORRELL, F., ROBERTS, L. and JASPER, H. H. 1956. Effect of focal epileptogenic lesions and their ablation upon conditioned electrical responses of the brain in the monkey. *Electroenceph. Clin. Neurophysiol.* 8:217-236.

MOTT, F. W. 1907. Bilateral lesion of the auditory cortical centre: complete deafness and aphasia. *Brit. Med. J.* pp. 310-315.

MOUTIER, F. 1908. *L'Aphasie de Broca*. Thèse, Paris. G. Steinheil, 687 pp.

MULLAN, J. and PENFIELD, W. 1959. Illusions of comparative interpretation and emotions produced by epileptic discharge and by electrical stimulation in temporal cortex. *Arch. Neurol. Psychiat.*, Chicago. (in press)

MUNK 1877. Cited by Head, H. 1926. Cambridge, University Press, p. 61.

NEEDLES, W. 1942. Concerning transfer of cerebral dominance in the function of speech. *J. Nerv. Ment. Dis.* 95:270-277.

NEWMAN, H. H. 1934. Dermatoglyphics and the problem of handedness. *Amer. J. Anat.* 55:277-321.

NIELSEN, J. M. 1936a. *Agnosia, Apraxia and Aphasia. Their Value in Cerebral Localization.* Los Angeles, The Los Angeles Neurological Society, 210 pp.

NIELSEN, J. M. 1936b. The possibility of pure motor aphasia. *Bull. Los Angeles Neurol. Soc.* 1:11-14.

NIELSEN, J. M. 1937. Unilateral cerebral dominance as related to mind blindness. *Arch. Neurol. Psychiat.*, Chicago. 38:108-135.

NIELSEN, J. M. 1939. The unsolved problems in aphasia. *Bull. Los Angeles Neurol. Soc.* 4:114-122.

NIELSEN, J. M. 1946. *Agnosia, Apraxia, Aphasia. Their Value in Cerebral Localization.* Ed. 2. New York, Paul B. Hoeber, Inc., 292 pp.

NIELSEN, J. M. 1948. The cortical motor pattern apraxias. *Res. Publ. Assoc. Nerv. Ment. Dis.* 27:565-581.

NIELSEN, J. M. 1953. Spontaneous recovery from aphasia: autopsy (report of a case). *Bull. Los Angeles Neurol. Soc.* 18:147-148.

NONNE 1899. Ein Fall von Aphasie. *Neurol. Zbl.* 18:1143-1144.

ODOM, G. L., DRATZ, H. M. and KRISTOFF, F. V. 1949. The effects of ultraviolet radiation on the exposed brain. Experimental study. *Ann. Surg.* 130:68-75.

ODOM, G. L. and LYMAN, R. S. 1946. Speech disorder following excision of postcentral gyrus. *Trans. Amer. Neurol. Assoc.* 71:67-70.

OGLE, W. 1867. Aphasia and agraphia. *St. George's Hosp. Rep.* 2:83-122.

OGLE, W. 1871. On dextral pre-eminence. *Med.-Chir. Trans.* 54:279-301.

OPPENHEIM, H. 1913. *Lehrbuch der Nervenkrankheiten.* Ed. 6. Berlin, S. Karger. Vol. II, pp. 951-973.

ORTON, S. T. 1934. Some studies in the language function. *Res. Publ. Assoc. Nerv. Ment. Dis.* 13:614-633.

ORTON, S. T. 1937. *Reading, Writing and Speech Problems in Children.* New York, W. W. Norton and Co., Inc., 215 pp.

PAGET, G. E. 1887. Notes on an exceptional case of aphasia. *Brit. Med. J.* pp. 1258-1259.

PENFIELD, W. 1930. Diencephalic autonomic epilepsy. *Res. Publ. Assoc. Nerv. Ment. Dis.* 9:645-663.

PENFIELD, W. 1938. The cerebral cortex in man: I. The cerebral cortex and consciousness. *Arch. Neurol. Psychiat.*, Chicago 40:417-442. Also in French, trans. by Professor H. Piéron in *L'Année Psychologique*, 1938. Vol. 39, 32 pp.

PENFIELD, W. 1947. Some observations of the cerebral cortex of man. Ferrier Lecture. *Proc. Roy. Soc. B.* 134:329-347.

PENFIELD, W. 1950. The supplementary motor area in the cerebral cortex of man. *Arch. Psychiat. Nervenkr.* 185:670-674.

PENFIELD, W. 1952. Epileptic automatism and the centrencephalic system. *Res. Publ. Assoc. Nerv. Ment. Dis.* 30:513-528.

PENFIELD, W. 1953. A consideration of the neurophysiological mechanisms of speech and some educational consequences. *Proc. Amer. Acad. Arts Sci.* 82:199-214.

PENFIELD, W. 1954a. Mechanisms of voluntary movements. *Brain* 77:1-17.

PENFIELD, W. 1954b. The permanent record of the stream of consciousness. *Proc. 14th. Internat. Congr. Psychol.* June, 1954, pp. 47-69.

PENFIELD, W. 1958a. *The Excitable Cortex in Conscious Man.* Fifth Sherrington Lecture. Liverpool, Liverpool University Press; Springfield, Ill. Charles C. Thomas, 42 pp.

PENFIELD, W. 1958b. Some mechanisms of consciousness discovered during electrical stimulation of the brain. *Proc. Nat. Acad. Sc.* 44:51-66.

PENFIELD, W. 1958c. Functional localization in temporal and deep Sylvian areas. *Res. Publ. Assoc. Nerv. Ment. Dis.* (1956) 36:210-226.

PENFIELD, W. and BOLDREY, E. 1937. Somatic motor and sensory representation in the cerebral cortex as studied by electrical stimulation. *Brain* 60:389-443.

PENFIELD, W. and HUMPHREYS, S. 1940. Epileptogenic lesions of the brain. A histologic study. *Arch. Neurol. Psychiat.*, Chicago. 43:240-261.

PENFIELD, W. and JASPER, H. 1947. Highest level seizures. *Res. Publ. Assoc. Nerv. Ment. Dis.* 26:252-271.

PENFIELD, W. and JASPER, H. H. 1954. *Epilepsy and the Functional Anatomy of the Human Brain.* Boston, Little, Brown and Co., 896 pp.

PENFIELD, W. and MILNER, B. 1958. Memory deficit produced by bilateral lesions in the hippocampal zone. *Arch. Neurol. Psychiat.*, Chicago 79:475-497.

PENFIELD, W. and PASQUET, A. 1954. Combined regional and general anaesthesia for craniotomy and cortical exploration. *Curr. Res. Anesth.* 33:145-164.

PENFIELD, W. and RASMUSSEN, T. 1949. Vocalization and arrest of speech. *Arch. Neurol. Psychiat.*, Chicago. 61:21-27.

PENFIELD, W. and RASMUSSEN, T. 1950. *The Cerebral Cortex of Man.* New York, The Macmillan Co., 235 pp.

PENFIELD, W. and WELCH, K. 1949. Instability of response to stimulation of the sensorimotor cortex of man. *J. Physiol.* 109:358-365.

PENFIELD, W. and WELCH, K. 1951. The supplementary motor area of the cerebral cortex. A clinical and experimental study. *Arch. Neurol. Psychiat.*, Chicago. 66:289-317.

PETIT-DUTAILLIS, D., CHRISTOPHE, J., PERTUISET, B., DREYFUS-BRISAC, C. and BLANC, C. 1954. Lobectomie temporale bilatérale pour épilepsie. Evolution des perturbations fonctionnelles postopératoires. *Rev. Neurol.* 91:129-133.

PETIT-DUTAILLIS, D., GUIOT, G., MESSIMY, R. and BOURDILLON, C. 1954.

A propos d'une aphémie par atteinte de la zone motrice supplémentaire de Penfield, au cours de l'évolution d'un anévrisme artério-veineux. Guérison de l'aphémie par ablation de la lésion. *Rev. Neurol.* 90:95-106.

PICK, A. 1892. Beiträge zur Lehre von den Sprachstörungen. *Arch. Psychiat. Nervenkr.* 23:896-918.

PICK, A. 1913. *Die agrammatischen Sprachstörungen.* Berlin, Julius Springer, cited by Head, 1926, 230 pp.

POPPEN, J. L. 1939. Ligation of the left anterior cerebral artery. Its hazards and means of avoidance of its complications. *Arch. Neurol. Psychiat.*, Chicago. 41:495-503.

PRADOS, M., STROWGER, B. and FEINDEL, W. H. 1945. Studies on cerebral edema. I. Reaction of the brain to air exposure; pathologic changes; II. Physiologic changes. *Arch. Neurol. Psychiat.*, Chicago. 54:163-174; 290-300.

PREOBRASHENSKI, P. A. 1893. Zur Pathologie des Gehirns. *Neurol. Zbl.* 12:759-760.

PREOBRASHENSKI, P. A. 1902. Zur Lehre von der subcorticalen Alexie und ähnlichen Störungen. *Neurol. Zbl.* 21:734-736.

PYE-SMITH, P. H. 1871. On left-handedness. *Guy's Hosp. Rep.*, 3rd. S. 16:141-146.

RAGGI 1915. Cited by Ardin-Delteil, Levi-Valensi and Derrieu, 1923.

RANEY, A. A., FRIEDMAN, A. P. and NIELSEN, J. M. 1942. Aphasia after major temporal lobectomy. *Bull. Los Angeles Neurol. Soc.* 7:154-156.

RASMUSSEN, T. and WADA, J. 1959. The intracarotid injection of sodium amytal for the lateralization of cerebral speech dominance: experimental and clinical observations. *J. Neurosurg.* (in press)

RAYMOND, F. and ARTAUD, G. 1884. Contribution à l'étude des localisations cérébrales (Trajet intra-cérébral de l'hypogosse). *Arch. Neurol.*, Paris. 7:145-172; 296-307.

RAYMOND, F. and DREYFOUS, F. 1882. Contribution à l'étude de l'aphasie. *Arch. Neurol.*, Paris. 3:80-86.

REINHOLD, M. 1950. A case of auditory agnosia. *Brain* 73:203-223.

REINHOLD, M. 1954. An analysis of agnosia. *Neurology* 4:128-136.

REITAN, R. M. 1953. Intellectual functions in aphasic and non-aphasic brain injured subjects. *Neurology* 3:202-212.

RIESE, W. 1947. The early history of aphasia. *Bull. Hist. Med.* 21:322-334.

RIESE, W. 1949. Aphasia in brain tumors. Its appearance in relation to the natural history of the lesion. *Confin. Neurol.*, Basel. 9:64-79.

RIESE, W. 1952. 7. Über Plastizität des Nervensystems, ihr Wesen, ihre Geschichte und ihre Anwendung in der Klinik. *Schweiz. Arch. Neurol. Psychiat.* 69:236-247.

RIESE, W. and HOFF, E. C. 1950. A history of the doctrine of cerebral localization: sources, anticipators and basic reasoning. *J. Hist. Med.* 5:50-71.

RIESEN, A. H. 1947. The development of visual perception in man and chimpanzee. *Science* 106:107-108.

RIFE, D. C. 1939. Handedness of twins. *Science* 89:178-179.

RIFE, D. C. 1941. Palm patterns and handedness. *Science* 94:187.

RIFE, D. C. 1951. Heredity and handedness. *Sci. Mon.*, New York. 73: 188-191.

RIFE, D. C. and KLOEPFER, H. W. 1943. An investigation of the linkage relationship of the blood groups and types with hand patterns and handedness. *Ohio J. Sci.* 43:182-185.

ROBB, J. P. 1946. *A Study of the Effects of Cortical Excision on Speech in Patients with Previous Cerebral Injuries.* M.Sc. Thesis, McGill University, Montreal, 121 pp.

ROBB, J. P. 1948. Effect of cortical excision and stimulation of the frontal lobe on speech. *Res. Publ. Assoc. Nerv. Ment. Dis.* 27:587-609.

ROBERTS, L. 1949. *A Study of Certain Alterations in Speech during Stimulation of Specific Cortical Regions.* M.Sc. Thesis, McGill University, Montreal, 117 pp.

ROBERTS, L. 1951. Alterations in speech produced by cerebral stimulation. *Trans. Amer. Neurol. Assoc.* 76:43-47.

ROBERTS, L. 1952. *Alterations in Speech Produced by Cerebral Stimulation and Excision.* Ph.D. Thesis, McGill University, Montreal, 239 pp.

ROBERTS, L. 1955. Handedness and Cerebral Dominance. *Trans. Amer. Neurol. Assoc.* 80:143-147.

ROBERTS, L. 1958a. Functional plasticity in cortical speech areas and the integration of speech. *Res. Publ. Assoc. Nerv. Ment. Dis.* (1956) 36:449-466 and *Arch. Neurol. Psychiat.*, Chicago, 79:275-283.

ROBERTS, L. 1958b. *Activation and Interference Produced by Electrical Stimulation of the Brain in Conscious Man.* Symposium on Brain Stimulation. Austin, Texas, Univ. of Texas Press, Sheer, D., Editor. (in press)

ROBERTS, L. 1958c. Dysphasias from the Neurological Standpoint. *Speech Pathology and Therapy.* Baltimore, Williams & Wilkins Co., Levin, M., Editor. (in press)

ROTHSCHILD, K. 1931. The relation of Broca's center to lefthandedness. *Amer. J. Med. Sci.* 182:116-118.

ROTHMAN, M. 1907. Zur Symptomatologie der Hemiplegie. *Neurol. Zbl.* 26:371-372.

ROTHMAN, M. 1909. Discussion of Stier, Erkennung und Bedeutung der Linkshändigkeit. *Zbl. Nervenheilk.* 32:718.

RUNEBURG 1896. *Finska Läkaresällskap handl.* 38:837-842. Extract in *Neurol. Zbl.*, 1898, 17:238.

RUSSELL, J. 1874. Note on a case of left hemiplegia with loss of speech occurring in a left-handed patient. *Med. Times and Gaz.*, London. 2:36, 47.

RYLE, G. 1950. In *The Physical Basis of Mind*. Laslett, P., Editor. Oxford, Blackwell, p. 75.

SACHS, B. 1905. *A Treatise on the Nervous Diseases of Children*. Ed. 2. New York, Wm. Wood, p. 439.

SCHEINKER, I. M. and KUHR, B. M. 1948. Motor aphasia and agraphia caused by small vascular lesion confined to third and second convolutions of left frontal lobe. *Res. Publ. Assoc. Nerv. Ment. Dis.* 27:582-586.

SCHILDER, Paul 1932. Localization of the body image (postural model of the body). *Res. Publ. Assoc. Nerv. Ment. Dis.* 13:466-484.

SCHILLER, F. 1947. Aphasia studied in patients with missile wounds. *J. Neurol. Psychiat.* 10:183-197.

SCHREIBER, J. 1874. Beitrag zur Lehre von der Aphasie. *Berlin Klin. Wochen.* 11:308-309; 320-322.

SCHUBERT, K. and PANSE, F. 1953. Audiologische Befunde bei sensorischer Aphasie. *Arch. Ohr-, Nas.-u. Kehlk Heilk.* 164:23-40.

SCHUELL, H. 1953. Aphasic difficulties understanding spoken language. *Neurology* 3:176-184.

SCHUELL, H. 1954. Clinical observations on aphasia. *Neurology* 4:179-189.

SCHUKNECHT, H. F. and WOELLNER, R. C. 1955. An experimental and clinical study of deafness from lesions of the cochlear nerve. *J. Laryng. Otol.* 49:75-97.

SEMMES, J. 1953. Agnosia in animal and man. *Psychol. Rev.* 60:140-147.

SEMMES, J. 1956. Personal communication to the author.

SEMMES, J., WEINSTEIN, S., GHENT, L. and TEUBER, H. L. 1954. Performance on complex tactual tasks after brain injury in man: Analysis by locus of lesion. *Amer. J. Psychol.* 67:220-240.

SEMMES, J., WEINSTEIN, S., GHENT, L. and TEUBER, H. L. 1955. Spatial orientation in man after cerebral injury: Analysis by locus of lesion. *J. Psychol.* 39:227-244.

SENATOR, H. 1904. Aphasie mit links-seitiger Hemiplegie bei Rechtshändigkeit. *Charité-Ann.* 28:150-158.

SENDEN, M. v. 1932. *Raum- und Gestaltenffassung bei operierten Blindgeborenen vor und nach der Operation*. Leipzig, Barth, 303 pp.

SHAW, E. A. 1893. The sensory side of aphasia. *Brain* 16:492-514.

SHERRINGTON, C. S. 1947. *The Integrative Action of the Nervous System*. Cambridge, University Press, pp. 274-276.

SINGER, H. D. and LOW, A. A. 1933a. The brain in a case of motor aphasia in which improvement occurred with training. *Arch. Neurol. Psychiat.*, Chicago. 29:162-165.

SINGER, H. D. and LOW, A. A. 1933b. Acalculia (Henschen). *Arch. Neurol. Psychiat.*, Chicago. 29:467-498.

SMITH, R. P. 1917-1918. Aphasia in relation to mental disease. *Proc. Roy. Soc. Med.* (neurol.) 11:1-20.

SMITH, S. and HOLMES, G. 1916. A case of bilateral motor apraxia with disturbance of visual orientation. *Brit. Med. J.* pp. 437-451.

SMITH, W. K. 1941. Vocalization and other responses elicited by excitation of the regio cingularis in the monkey. *Amer. J. Physiol.* 133:451-452.

SMYTH, G. E. and STERN, K. 1938. Tumours of the thalamus—A clinico-pathological study. *Brain* 61:339-374.

SOUQUES, A. 1910. Aphasie avec hémiplégie gauche chez un droitier. *Rev. Neurol.* 2:547-549.

SOUQUES, A. 1928. Quelques cas d'anarthrie de Pierre Marie. *Rev. Neurol.* 2:319-368.

SPALKE 1927. Cited by Ludwig, 1938.

SPENCER, H. 1892. *The Principles of Psychology.* New York, Appleton, 2 vols.

SPILLER, W. G. 1906. Lesions of the left first temporal convolution in relation to sensory aphasia. *Rev. Neurol. Psychiat.* 4:329-338.

STARR, M. A. 1889. The pathology of sensory aphasia, with an analysis of fifty cases in which Broca's centre was not diseased. *Brain* 12:82-101.

STAUFFENBERG v. 1918. Klinische und anatomische Beiträge zur Kenntnis der aphasischen, agnostischen und apraktischen Symptome. *Z. ges. Neurol. Psychiat.* 39:71-212.

STONE, L. 1934. Paradoxical symptoms in right temporal lobe tumor. *J. Nerv. Ment. Dis.* 79:1-13.

SUBIRANA, A. 1952. La droiterie. *Schweiz. Arch. Neurol. Psychiat.* 69:321-359.

SUBIRANA, A. 1956. 1. Vision neurologique des troubles du langage d'intérêt phoniatrique: Le pronostic des aphasies de l'adulte. *Folia Phoniatr.*, Basel. 8:147-197.

SUBIRANA, A., COROMINAS, J., PUNCERNAU, R., OLLER-DAURELLA, L. and MONTEYS, J. 1952. Neuva contribución al estudio de la dominancia cerebral. *Medicamenta*, Madrid. 10:255-258.

SUTER, C. 1953. Anomic aphasia: differential diagnosis and cerebral localization of lesion in 20 cases. *J. Amer. Med. Assoc.* 151:462-468.

SYMONDS, C. 1953. Aphasia. *J. Neurol. Psychiat.* 16:1-6.

TATERKA, H. 1924. Partielle Apraxie des rechten Armes nach linksseitiger Hemiplegie bei einer Linkshänderin. *Z. ges. Neurol. Psychiat.* 90:573-579.

TAYLOR, F. 1880. Right hemiplegia after scarlatina, with embolism of the middle cerebral artery, destruction of Broca's convolution without aphasia, and death from diphtheria. *Med. Times & Gaz.* p. 686.

TEITELBAUM, H. A. 1943. An analysis of the disturbances of the higher cortical functions, agnosia, apraxia and aphasia. *J. Nerv. Ment. Dis.* 97:44-61.

TEMKIN, O. 1945. *The Falling Sickness.* Baltimore, Johns Hopkins University Press, 380 pp.

TEUBER, H. L. and BENDER, M. B. 1948. Critical flicker frequency in defective fields of vision. *Fed. Proc.* 7:123-124.

TILNEY, F. 1936. Discussion of Kennedy, F. and Wolf, A. Relationship of intellect to speech in patients with aphasia, with illustrative cases. *Arch. Neurol. Psychiat.*, Chicago. 36:897-898.

TISON, E. 1889. Hémiplégie gauche avec aphasie; insuffisance de la valvule mitrale avec rétrécissement de l'orifice; sarcome lipomateux de l'ovaire droit. *Bull. Soc. Anat.*, Paris. 64:570-573.

TOUCHE 1899. Contribution a l'étude clinique et anatomopathologique de l'aphasie sensorielle. *Arch. Gén. Méd.* S. 9, 2:640-660.

TROUSSEAU 1865. Discussion sur la faculté du langage articulé. *Bull. Acad. Méd.* 30:647-675.

USTVEDT, H. J. 1937. Ueber die Untersuchung der musikalischen Funktionen bei Patienten mit Gehirnleiden, besonders bei Patienten mit Aphasie. *Acta Med. Scandinav.* Suppl. 86, 737 pp.

WADA, J. 1949. A new method for the determination of the side of cerebral speech dominance: A preliminary report on the intracarotid injection of sodium amytal in man. *Med. Biol.* 14:221-222.

WADHAM, W. 1869. Aphasia. *St. George's Hosp. Rep.* 4:245-250.

WALKER, A. E. 1938a. *The Primate Thalamus.* Chicago, University of Chicago Press, 321 pp.

WALKER, A. E. 1938b. The thalamus of the chimpanzee. IV. Thalamic projections to the cerebral cortex. *J. Anat.* 73:37-93.

WARREN, J. M. 1953. Handedness in the rhesus monkey. *Science* 118:622-623.

WEBER, E. 1904. Das Schreiben als Ursache der einseitigen Lage des Sprachzentrums. *Zbl. Physiol.* 18:341-347.

WECHSLER, L. S. 1937. Excision of the speech area without resultant aphasia. *Arch. Neurol. Psychiat.*, Chicago. 38:430-437.

WEISENBURG, T. and McBRIDE, K. E. 1935. *Aphasia. A Clinical and Psychological Study.* New York, The Commonwealth Fund; Brattleboro, Vt., E. L. Hildred & Co., 634 pp.

WELCH, K. and PENFIELD, W. 1950. Paradoxical improvement in hemiplegia following cortical excision. *J. Neurosurg.* 7:414-420.

WEPMAN, J. P. 1951. *Recovery from Aphasia.* New York, The Ronald Press Co., 263 pp.

WERNICKE, C. 1874. *Der aphasische Symptomencomplex.* Breslau, Max Cohn and Weigert, 72 pp.

WESTPHAL 1884. Ueber einem Fall von Tumor des linken Schläfenlappens. *Neurol. Zbl.* 3:21-22.

WHITE, H. 1887. Left hemiplegia and hemianaesthesia, and aphasia and left-sided apraxia in a left-handed woman. *Brit. Med. J.* p. 675.

WILSON, S. A. K. 1908. A contribution to the study of apraxia with a review of the literature. *Brain* 31:164-216.

WILSON, S. A. K. 1920. Discussion on aphasia. *Brain* 43:433-438.

WILSON, S. A. K. 1926. *Aphasia.* London, Kegan Paul, Trench, Trubner & Co., 109 pp.

WOHLFART, G., LINDGREN, A. and JERNELIUS, B. 1952. Clinical picture and morbid anatomy in a case of "pure word deafness." *J. Nerv. Ment. Dis.* 116:818-827.

WOOD, H. C. 1889. Right-sided aphasia in a left-handed person. *Med. News.* 54:484-485.

ZANGWILL, O. L. 1951. Discussion on parietal lobe syndromes. *Proc. Roy. Soc. Med.* 44:337-346.

ZANGWILL, O. L. 1954. Agraphia due to a left parietal glioma in left-handed man. *Brain* 77:510-520.

ZIEGLER, D. K. 1952. Word deafness and Wernicke's aphasia. *Arch. Neurol. Psychiat.*, Chicago. 67:323-331.

ZOLLINGER, R. 1935. Removal of the left cerebral hemisphere. Report of a case. *Arch. Neurol. Psychiat.*, Chicago. 34:1055-1064.

ZUCKER, K. 1934. An analysis of disturbed function in aphasia. *Brain* 57:109-127.

CASE INDEX

A. D.

~~~~~~

A

A.Ay. 175, 176
P.A. 156, 158

B

A.Bra. 52
M.Bu. 34

C

J.Ch. 163, 164

D

A.Do. 145, 146, 184, 221
D.Da. 154, 156

F

D.F. 52
G.F. 51
M.F. 169, 170

H

C.H. 111, 113-116, 138, 227, 228, 231
D.Ha. 161, 162, 180

J

C.J. 174, 175
L.Jo. 159, 161

K

A.K. 177

L

E.L. 154, 155
E.Ls. 172, 173

M

J.Ma. 151, 152, 184, 222
J.Mc. 165, 166
J.Mo. 148, 149, 224
M.Ma. 45, 46, 47
T.M. 169, 171, 222
W.My. 177, 178

N

H.N. 167, 168, 184

O

W.Oe. 143, 144, 224

P

H.Py. 35
W.Pe. 148, 150, 224

R

J.Rl. 150, 151
P.Rx. 159, 160

S

M.St. 215
T.S. 52

T

J.T. 50

V

J.V. 34

Y

C.Y. 142, 185

GENERAL INDEX

A. D.